WHY YOU CAN'T LOSE WEIGHT

WHY IT'S SO HARD TO SHED POUNDS AND WHAT YOU CAN DO ABOUT IT

PAMELA WARTIAN SMITH, MD, MPH

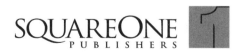

SQUAREONE
PUBLISHERS

EDITOR: Joanne Abrams, Marie Caratozzolo, Colleen Day, and Michael Weatherhead
COVER DESIGNER: Jeannie Tudor
TYPESETTER: Gary A. Rosenberg

The information and advice contained in this book are based upon the research and the personal and professional experiences of the author. They are not intended as a substitute for consulting with a health-care professional. The publisher and author are not responsible for any adverse effects or consequences resulting from the use of any of the suggestions or procedures discussed in this book. All matters pertaining to your physical health should be supervised by a health-care professional. It is a sign of wisdom, not cowardice, to seek a second or third opinion.

Square One Publishers
115 Herricks Road
Garden City Park, NY 11040
(516) 535-2010 • (877) 900-BOOK
www.squareonepublishers.com

Library of Congress Cataloging-in-Publication Data

Smith, Pamela Wartian.
  Why you can't lose weight : why it's so hard to shed pounds and what you can do about it / Pamela Wartian Smith.
     p. cm.
  Includes bibliographical references and index.
  ISBN 978-0-7570-0312-7 (pbk.)
  1. Weight loss—Popular works. I. Title.
  RM222.2.S62295 2011
  613.2'5—dc22
                              2011007030

Printed in Canada

10   9   8   7   6   5   4   3   2   1

Contents

Part III Biochemical Factors

Part IV Solutions

To my patients, whom I have had the blessing to serve all of these years.

Acknowledgments

I would like to thank my publisher, Rudy Shur, without whom this book would not be possible. His belief in my message was instrumental in making this book the best it can be.

I would also like to thank my project editor, Joanne Abrams, for her hard work and dedication, and Square One editors Marie Caratozzolo, Colleen Day, and Michael Weatherhead, who all made important contributions to the book.

Introduction

I f you have tried time and again to lose weight, you know how frustrating it can be. You try diet after diet. You restrict calories, perhaps limit your consumption of a specific food group like carbohydrates or fats, and still those stubborn pounds remain. But the truth is that successful weight loss does not depend solely on what you put in your mouth. Yes, calories consumed should equal calories burned, but many more factors are involved in the process of putting weight on and the process of taking it off. That's why this book was written. Based on the latest information on why people gain weight and why they have so much trouble losing it, *Why You Can't Lose Weight* fills you in on the many factors, from lifestyle issues to hormonal dysfunction, that may be stopping you from successfully dropping pounds. More importantly, it guides you in treating these problems so that you can improve your lifestyle, enhance your overall health, and finally succeed at weight loss. There are very real reasons—beyond calorie intake—that can cause weight gain. Here, for the first time, is a book that helps you understand and identify these reasons and steer a true course to weight-loss success.

Why You Can't Lose Weight begins by providing basic information about how your body deals with food. Why does your body burn some of the food you eat as energy and store some of it as fat? What makes you hungry in the first place? Chapter 1 answers these questions to provide a clear picture of what's going on inside your body.

Part I of *Why You Can't Lose Weight* looks at lifestyle practices that can frustrate your attempts to lose weight. Exercise, fiber intake, sleep, and water are all crucial to the weight-loss process. If you neglect any of these important elements, it becomes more difficult to stick to or benefit from even the healthiest of diets. Stress can also affect weight, as can food addictions. Each chapter in Part I examines one of these issues so that you can understand it, recognize it, and adopt healthy lifestyle practices that will contribute to a healthy weight.

A number of health disorders, too, can cause you to gain weight and make it difficult to shed pounds. Part II targets several common problems that can contribute to excess weight, including food allergies, chronic inflammation, thyroid hormone dysfunction (hypothyroidism), toxic buildup, and chronic yeast infections. You will learn what these conditions are, how you and your health-care providers can detect them, and how you can take steps toward not only the relief of symptoms, but also a healthier, slimmer body.

To lose weight, your body must produce and appropriately respond to thousands of important biochemicals, such as estrogen, insulin, and serotonin. That's what Part III is all about. Each chapter looks at a biochemistry-related problem, including depression, female hormone imbalance, insulin resistance, male hormone insufficiency, and neurotransmitter (brain chemical) dysfunction. Also included is information on how your genetic makeup can influence the way you gain and lose weight. Again, you'll learn how these disorders can be recognized, how they affect your body, and what you can do to restore a healthy biochemical balance and body weight.

For each problem discussed, *Why You Can't Lose Weight* tells you about the different approaches you can take to greater health. For instance, if chronic inflammation is preventing you from shedding weight, you can eliminate inflammatory foods from your diet, take anti-inflammatory nutritional supplements, and use a moderate exercise program to normalize your body's inflammatory response. If this multilevel strategy sounds a little overwhelming, turn to Chapter 20, "Putting It All Together." Here, you'll discover vital information on selecting and following a healthy diet, choosing and using supplements, and setting up a safe and effective exercise routine, all with the goal of creating a customized, easy-to-follow weight-loss plan. You'll also learn a little more about some of the professionals who can provide further information, guidance, and support. The "Resources" section, which begins on page 207, offers additional assistance by filling you in on diagnostic laboratories, supplement companies, and professional organizations—everything you need to know to work towards a slimmer you.

As you read through this book to pinpoint the cause of your weight problem, keep in mind that the body is a complex piece of machinery and that its many functions are interrelated. For this reason, there may be more than one factor that is undermining your efforts to lose weight. For instance, low thyroid function, covered in Chapter 10, may cause depression, which is addressed in Chapter 13. You have to treat both problems if you want to feel better and reach your desired weight. Fortunately, several of the get-well strategies discussed in the book—regular exercise and a healthy diet, for instance—are useful in relieving a range of problems. Nevertheless, if you treat one disorder and find that you are still unable to lose weight, it makes sense to read the remaining chapters to learn if other factors may be at work. A good way to start your detective work is to take the self-test that appears at the beginning of each of the first three parts. (See pages 13, 63, and 113.) Once you complete each test and review your scores, you will have a clearer idea of whether your weight problems are caused by lifestyle habits, health disorders, biochemical dysfunctions, or, perhaps, a combination of these factors.

I don't have to tell you how dangerous excess weight can be. Being overweight or obese increases the risk for thirty-five major diseases, including diabetes, heart disease, stroke, arthritis, sleep apnea, and cancer. Excess weight has such an impact on health that recently, the National Research Council cited obesity as one of the chief reasons why life expectancy for Americans lags well behind that of other developed nations—even though we spend more money on health care than any other country.

If you have tried one-size-fits-all weight-loss plans only to find that those added pounds simply won't go away, it's time to learn exactly what's keeping you from shedding those pounds. With *Why You Can't Lose Weight*, you'll discover how to lose weight, keep it off, and enjoy radiant health.

1

What Really Goes on Inside Your Body?

This book explores the many factors, from food allergies to inadequate water consumption, that can frustrate your attempts to diet successfully. But before you can understand the reasons why your body may be holding onto excess weight, it's useful to know the basics of how the body normally deals with food. What makes you hungry? What happens to your food once you chew and swallow it? And why, under certain circumstances, is some of it stored as fat? That's what this chapter is all about. It begins by briefly looking at why you eat, and then explains what your body does with the food both during the digestive process and afterwards.

WHY DO YOU GET HUNGRY?

On the surface, it seems simple. When you are hungry, you eat. But what causes the feeling of hunger? Understanding why you feel the need to eat can help you to understand the processes of weight gain and loss.

When your stomach and intestines are empty, they produce chemicals which signal the brain that your body needs food. Two hormones that affect your appetite are *ghrelin,* which makes you feel hungry, and *leptin,* which lets you know you are full. When your stomach is empty, you make more ghrelin and less leptin, and this combination stimulates the feeling of hunger.

It is also possible to experience false hunger. If you have gone for some time without eating, your mind may perceive that your body should be hungry when it really is not. If you are accustomed to eating at certain times each day, your mind may think you should be eating at that time, even if your body doesn't really need nourishment. If you see or smell delicious food, you may think that you are hungry even if you have just

5

eaten. This is the most powerful kind of false hunger, since your senses are developed specifically to drive you towards food that is appetizing.

HOW DOES DIGESTION WORK?

Let's say that in response to your hunger, you eat a turkey sandwich with lettuce and mayonnaise. What happens to the food? It enters the digestive tract.

The digestive tract is made of a series of hollow organs connected together in a long, winding tube. From top to bottom, the tract includes the mouth, esophagus, stomach, small intestine, large intestine (also known as the colon), rectum, and anus. These organs contain smooth muscle that breaks down food and moves it forward inside the body. The digestive system also includes the liver and the pancreas, which produce their own digestive juices, and the gallbladder, which stores the liver's juices until they are needed in the small intestine.

In order for the body to use the nutrients in the food you eat, that food needs to be broken down into the smallest useable parts. Digestion starts in the mouth, where food is chewed and mixed with saliva to make it soft enough to pass through the digestive tract. Saliva also contains proteins called *enzymes*, which begin to chemically break down carbohydrates—like the bread in your sandwich—into simple sugar molecules. The chewed ball of food, called a *bolus*, is swallowed and enters the esophagus, after which involuntary muscles move the bolus down to the stomach.

In the stomach, digestive juices and muscle contractions work on the food to break it down. *Gastric acid*, produced in the stomach, does the most work here by weakening the chemical bonds between molecules of food. Carbohydrates are the simplest foods and the easiest to digest, and therefore spend the least amount of time in the stomach. Proteins, such as the turkey in your sandwich, are slightly larger molecules and take longer to dissolve in the acid. Because fats, found in the mayonnaise on your bread, are the most complex molecules, they sit in the stomach the longest. In fact, fats are not fully digested when they leave the stomach, but finish being digested in the small intestine.

The food slowly moves into the small intestine, where digestion continues as the food is pushed along. Glands in the small intestine are activated when the organ's walls are stretched by the food, and intestinal juices are produced. These juices finish breaking down the food and, along with juices from the pancreas, neutralize the stomach acid so that it does not damage the rest of the digestive tract. Bile from the liver is added to digest fats. The gallbladder stores bile until food is present, and then empties it into the small intestine. Similar to how dish soap removes grease stuck to a cooking pan, bile surrounds and dissolves fat into molecules small enough to be completely broken down by the intestinal and pancreatic juices.

When all is said and done, carbohydrates, proteins, and fats are finally reduced to their basic molecular components as they travel through the small intestine. Carbohydrates turn into simple sugars like *glucose* and *fructose*, which are needed for energy. Proteins become generic building blocks called *amino acids*, which are used to repair tissues and build new cells. Fats are separated into *fatty acids* and *glycerols*, which contain far more energy than sugars and can either be used right away, or changed into other forms and stored. But how do these crucial components get to the cells that need them? Lining the walls of the small intestine are tiny finger-like projections called *villi*. Villi are designed to increase the surface area of the small intestine so that specialized cells can absorb nutrients into the bloodstream. Once in the bloodstream, nutrients are carried all over the body, where they pass through cell walls and are used for life functions.

Not all material can be absorbed. The romaine lettuce on that sandwich contains many necessary vitamins and minerals, but the majority of the plant matter is *fiber*, an indigestible material that cannot be taken in by the body. Fiber and old cells are pushed into the large intestine, where excess water and salts are absorbed back into the body to be reused. Certain bacteria in the large intestine also help digest some of the carbohydrates your body is unable to break down alone. These carbohydrates are absorbed here, along with nutrients like vitamin K, calcium, and iron. The remaining waste is stored in the rectum until it is eliminated through a bowel movement.

After you finish digesting your sandwich, your body will eventually signal the brain that you are hungry again. How quickly this happens depends on a number of factors, such as when and how fast you eat, how many calories you consume, the amount of exercise you do, how much fiber is in your diet, and how much water you drink. Several of these factors will be discussed in detail in later chapters. (See Chapter 2 to learn about exercise, Chapter 3 for a discussion of fiber, and Chapter 7 for information on water.)

HOW AND WHEN IS FAT STORED BY THE BODY?

In the earlier pages of this chapter, you learned that after your food is digested, nutrients are delivered to the body's cells, where they are absorbed and used. But not all nutrients are immediately utilized by the body; some are stored as fat. The reason for this dates back millions of years. In prehistoric times, food was far more difficult to obtain and store all year round, so humans would go through periods of plenty followed by periods of famine. Fat evolved in order to save energy in the body for those times of famine. Now, when getting dinner is no more complicated than a trip to the grocery store or a local fast food restaurant, Americans rarely go through the kind of food deprivation that calls for the use of reserves, but the process of storing fat hasn't disappeared.

What Are the Primary Factors That Affect Your Metabolic Rate?

Your metabolic rate is affected by numerous factors. Some, such as age, are beyond your control, while others, such as exercise, are yours to change. Below, I've listed the most common factors that influence metabolic rate.

- *Age.* Metabolism peaks during late adolescence, between ages fifteen to eighteen for women and eighteen to twenty-one for men. As you age, it slows by about 3 percent every year.

- *Gender.* On average, men are physically larger and have more muscle mass than women. For this reason, a man's metabolic rate can be as much as 30 percent higher than a woman's.

- *Race.* African Americans tend to have a slower metabolic rate on average than Caucasian Americans. There may be differences among other ethnicities and races as well, but more studies are needed.

- *Climate.* Warmer weather lowers your metabolic rate because you spend less energy keeping yourself warm.

- *State of consciousness.* For most of the time you are asleep, your brain slows your bodily functions, such as heartbeat, breathing, and digestion. Since you are lying still for five to nine consecutive hours, far less energy is needed, so metabolic rate decreases.

As you learned earlier, different kinds of nutrients are digested at different rates. Carbohydrates finish dissolving first, and therefore enter the bloodstream most quickly for use as energy. This raises your blood sugar level, and the body uses *insulin,* the hormone produced by the pancreas, to change glucose into *glycogen,* which is stored in the liver and muscles. The amount of glycogen your body holds, however, is not very large—all your body's glycogen wouldn't even get you through one particularly active day. When your liver and muscles have enough glycogen stored, your body turns the remaining glycogen into fat molecules that are stored in fat cells. Any proteins not needed for cell repair are turned into sugars and, eventually, fats as well. The last nutrient, fat, is burned for energy or converted to substances like cholesterol. Any fat that is not immediately used is stored in fat cells for future use.

- *Size.* Heavier individuals actually have higher metabolic rates because they have more body mass for which they must provide energy.

- *Physical condition.* Fit people with a lean body composition have higher resting metabolic rates. A pound of muscle burns six times more energy than a pound of fat.

- *Exercise.* When you exercise, your metabolism speeds up to burn the energy needed to fuel your activity. It then remains elevated for twelve hours. Physical activity—especially if it includes strength training—also builds muscle mass, and as you already know, muscle is an efficient burner of fat.

- *Hormones.* Hormone levels in the body can affect metabolism, especially for women. Changes in estrogen and progesterone production—such as just before ovulation, during menstruation, and during menopause—can lower metabolic rates and lead to weight gain. Men produce certain amounts of these hormones, too, and are also susceptible to altered metabolic rates, particularly when experiencing lowered testosterone levels. (See Chapter 14 to learn about female hormones, and Chapter 17 to learn about male hormones.)

- *Stimulants.* Caffeine and nicotine use raises your heart rate and therefore temporarily increases metabolism. Alcohol, on the other hand, slows metabolism.

For men, the majority of fat cells are located on the chest, abdomen, and buttocks. Women store most of their fat cells in the hips, breasts, waist, and buttocks. About 10 percent of your fat cells die every year, but an equal number of new ones are produced to replace them. Nearly all fat molecules are stored in existing fat cells, which increase or decrease in size as necessary.

You are probably already aware that the amount of food your body stores as fat is affected by your *metabolism*—the transformation of food into the energy needed to fuel life processes. In America, the energy contained in food is measured in units called *calories*. If the amount of fuel needed to keep your body running is equal to the amount of fuel you take in, you are at a metabolic equilibrium and your weight will generally stay the same. For instance, if your body needs 2,000 calories of energy daily to run, consuming 2,000 calories in food and drink over the course of the day will provide this with little trouble. When you take in more fuel than you need—2,500 calories, for example—the extra is stored as fat, so you gain weight. Following this logic, you would think that by taking in less fuel than you need would result in losing weight, but this is not always the case. For one thing, the kind of calories you consume can influence whether or not fat is stored. The 500 calories found in a meal of fruits and vegetables is much harder to store as fat than 500 calories of French fries—and is more nutritious as well! In addition, when you go for long periods of time without eating, your body thinks it is being starved. Like the body of a prehistoric human, your body reacts to the possibility of famine by slowing metabolism to conserve energy and calories. A slower metabolism makes it much harder to burn the fat you already have, since your body is holding on to it "just in case." Fortunately, there is much you can do to increase your metabolism so that both the calories you take in and your stored body fat are burned more efficiently.

You now understand how the body processes food and uses it for energy or storage. The chief principle is fairly simple—calories consumed should be less than calories burned if you want to lose weight. Everyone is different, however, and there are a multitude of factors that can influence your ability to digest and absorb nutrients, metabolize food, and store or burn fat. Chapters 2 through 19 examine some of these factors so that you understand how your lifestyle or certain health disorders may be affecting your ability to achieve a healthy weight.

PART I

Lifestyle

Introduction
to Part I

The way you live your life absolutely affects the state of your health. Studies have shown that smart lifestyle practices contribute to a greater resistance to health disorders, an enhanced sense of well-being, and a slimmer, stronger body. Poor habits, on the other hand, open the door to a wide range of problems, from cancer and diabetes to weight gain and obesity.

Part I takes a close look at six lifestyle issues that have been linked to weight problems. Insufficient exercise, low fiber intake, food addictions, sleep deprivation, stress, and the inadequate consumption of water have all been shown not only to lead to weight gain, but also to make it difficult to lose excess pounds. In each chapter, you'll learn about the problem being examined, read about its symptoms, discover how this lifestyle habit can lead to weight gain, and find guidelines for determining if this problem is compromising your own health. Finally, you'll discover how you can modify your daily activities with the goal of achieving and maintaining a healthy weight as well as greater overall wellness.

All of us, at one time or another, have found ourselves skimping on sleep, grabbing a cup of coffee or a can of soda instead of a glass of pure water, or making other choices that can lead to the addition of unwanted pounds. The good news is that it is just as easy to make good lifestyle decisions as it is to make poor ones. If you're wondering if lifestyle factors are hindering your attempts to lose weight, take the self-test on page 13. If your answers indicate that these factors may be a problem, Chapters 2 through 7 will guide you in taking the first steps toward a healthier, slimmer body.

LIFESTYLE QUESTIONNAIRE

This test was designed to help you determine if lifestyle issues, such as lack of exercise or insufficient sleep, may be hindering your attempts to lose weight. For each of the following questions, check the box that most accurately applies to you. When you have completed the questionnaire, count the number of times you answered "Often." If you checked this answer more than ten times, chances are that your lifestyle is compromising your ability to lose unwanted pounds. Read Chapters 2 through 7 to learn why your answers may indicate a problem, and how simple changes in everyday habits and activities can help you lose weight.

	Seldom	Sometimes	Often
1. Do everyday activities, such as walking up a flight of stairs or lifting a box, cause you to become out of breath?	☐	☐	☐
2. Do you feel tired and sluggish during the day?	☐	☐	☐
3. Do you have trouble getting to sleep or wake up several times during the night?	☐	☐	☐
4. Do you feel sore and achy the day after doing any kind of physical activity?	☐	☐	☐
5. Do you eat a lot of processed or fast food, or foods high in protein and low in carbohydrates?	☐	☐	☐
6. Do you experience bloating, abdominal cramps, or upset stomach after eating?	☐	☐	☐
7. Are you hungry only an hour or two after eating?	☐	☐	☐
8. Do you obsessively think about food or experience cravings for certain foods that ultimately lead to binges?	☐	☐	☐
9. Do you feel out of control when you are eating?	☐	☐	☐

	Seldom	Sometimes	Often
10. Do you have trouble focusing on work or simple tasks?	☐	☐	☐
11. When you are sitting still for an extended period of time, do you catch yourself drifting off to sleep?	☐	☐	☐
12. Are you quick to snap at friends, family, and coworkers?	☐	☐	☐
13. Do you drink several cups of coffee or other caffeine-containing beverages throughout the day?	☐	☐	☐
14. Do you experience racing thoughts and the feeling of being overwhelmed?	☐	☐	☐
15. Do you lack focus and concentration when it comes to doing work or other daily tasks?	☐	☐	☐
16. Have you experienced chest, muscle, or stomach pain as a result of feeling pressured?	☐	☐	☐
17. Do you eat to deal with emotions like stress or depression rather than out of true physical need?	☐	☐	☐
18. Do you suffer from skin problems such as acne or dry skin?	☐	☐	☐
19. Does your daily fluid intake consist of mainly juice, soda, coffee, and/or tea?	☐	☐	☐
20. Is your urine dark yellow in color?	☐	☐	☐
TOTALS	_____	_____	_____

2

Insufficient Exercise

Sometimes, even your best efforts to eat healthy, consume the recommended amounts of fiber and water, and get eight hours of sleep each night will not result in weight loss. Why? The reason may have to do with your level of physical activity, or, as is more often the case, *inactivity*. An average day for many people goes something like this: You eat breakfast, get in a car, bus, or train to go to work, and sit at a desk for several hours. You temporarily leave your desk to eat a reasonable lunch, and then you return to your desk until it's time for your evening commute. After dinner, your night is spent unwinding by watching TV or reading, and, occasionally, eating a light snack. You may not be overeating, mindlessly snacking, or even eating the wrong foods—but you are not *moving* either.

The fact of the matter is that we live in an increasingly sedentary society, since modern technology and longer hours at desk jobs have made it less necessary (and less convenient) to be physically active. The annual National Health Interview Survey found that only 35 percent of adults over the age of eighteen engage in some kind of physical activity on a regular basis. A staggering one-third of adults do not engage in any activity at all. These statistics reflect the alarming—and rising—rates of obesity, diabetes, and heart disease in the country, not to mention high blood pressure and high cholesterol. Furthermore, they point to a likely reason why you, like so many other individuals, are unable to lose weight and keep it off. Decades of research have established a clear link between exercise and weight loss, so raising the level of physical activity among a progressively overweight population is of primary importance and concern.

WHAT IS EXERCISE?

There is an important distinction between physical activity and exercise. *Physical activity* is a general term that can be applied to any movement that engages the muscles, ranging from daily chores such as gardening, making beds, or vacuuming, to rigorous sports like tennis, running, or swimming, which raise the heart rate and build endurance. The term *exercise*, however, refers to planned, purposeful movement specifically intended to boost physical fitness. Running, walking, biking, swimming, sports, yoga, and dance are all activities that require effort, expend energy, and work core muscle groups.

Exercise is divided into two main categories, aerobic and anaerobic. *Aerobic exercise* (which is also called cardiovascular exercise) includes any activity that is rhythmic, continuous, and prolonged, and therefore increases your heart rate and requires additional intake of oxygen. Running, cycling, swimming, skating, aerobic dancing, climbing stairs, and jumping rope are all forms of aerobic exercise. *Anaerobic exercise,* on the other hand, requires very little increase in oxygen, as it is typically shorter in duration and of higher intensity. Weight lifting, sprinting, jumping, rowing, doing push-ups, doing sit-ups, and serving volleyballs or tennis balls are all examples of anaerobic exercise. These activities are generally more strenuous, involve quick bursts of energy, and result in muscle fatigue rather than an oxygen deficit.

Although anaerobic exercise builds strength and lean muscle, aerobic exercise is what health organizations like the American College of Sports Medicine (ACSM) are generally referring to when they give their recommendations for physical activity. According to the ACSM, American Health Association, and Surgeon General, adults need about thirty minutes of moderately intense cardiovascular activity (aerobic exercise) five days a week, or twenty minutes of vigorous cardiovascular activity three days a week.

WHAT ARE THE SYMPTOMS OF INSUFFICIENT EXERCISE?

The physical indicators of insufficient exercise go beyond just weight gain, and have just as much to do with how you feel as how you look. Some of the symptoms associated with lack of physical activity include:

- Knee pain

- Lack of mobility

- Loss of balance, especially in the elderly

- Loss of flexibility

- Low self-esteem

- Muscle strain

- Poor muscle tone

- Proneness to injury

- Sleep apnea and other sleep disorders

- Susceptibility to depression or anxiety

- Weakened immune system

If a number of these symptoms sound familiar to you, insufficient exercise may be a contributing factor to your weight loss problems.

HOW DOES EXERCISE CONTRIBUTE TO WEIGHT LOSS?

Exercise is a key element in any program designed to reduce weight and keep it off. Researchers at Princeton University have determined that exercise plays an important role in weight loss for several reasons. According to their findings, exercise:

- Activates the sympathetic nervous system, which regulates body functions such as the burning of fat.

- Boosts metabolism, thereby allowing your body to use and burn off calories at a quicker rate.

- Burns fat while maintaining lean muscle.

- Enhances insulin sensitivity.

- Releases the growth hormone, which facilitates weight loss and fortifies the body against aging and injury.

- Stimulates the activation of fat-burning brown fat (as opposed to white adipose tissue, which stores fat).

In sum, exercise triggers certain body functions and systems that aid the weight-loss process. Exercise burns excess calories that would otherwise be stored as fat, and it keeps your body's insulin levels in check, which in turn prevents energy deficits and weight gain.

Although it has been often argued that calorie reduction is more important than exercise when it comes to losing weight, weight loss cannot be *sustained* unless physical activity is incorporated into a weight-management program. To lose weight, you must burn more calories than you consume, and exercise is the most efficient way to ensure that this objective is met. By walking at a moderate pace for just thirty minutes a day, you can burn off a latte, half of a sandwich, or a small bag of potato chips. Cleaning your house for an hour can burn off even more calories, and swimming or running for the same length of time can potentially shave off an entire meal. Even when you're done exercising, your body will continue to burn calories and release energy, and the lean muscle you build through exercise is a natural—and perpetual—calorie-burner.

HOW DO YOU DETERMINE IF YOU ARE GETTING ENOUGH EXERCISE?

The amount of exercise needed to maintain a healthy weight and improve your well-being varies according to your weight and level of physical fitness. Generally speaking, you can assess your fitness level by paying attention to how you feel after engaging in physical activity. For instance, if you are out of breath after walking up a flight of stairs, frequently experience muscle tension, or become shaky and fatigued after only a few minutes of exercise, it's clear that you are out of shape.

The solution is to move more and make sure you do enough calorie-burning activities each day. It's possible to calculate your activity level in an average day by keeping track of the calories you burn doing various exercises or everyday activities like mowing the lawn, cleaning your kitchen, or sitting at your desk. When you consider this total alongside your caloric intake, you can figure out if your activity level is appropriate.

WHAT CAN YOU DO TO LOSE WEIGHT?

In order to lose 1 pound of body fat, you must burn 3,500 calories *in addition* to the number you are already burning in the course of your usual activities. This means that to lose 1 pound a week, you would have to eliminate 500 calories every day through calorie reduction, exercise, or both. Burning off five hundred calories, about the equivalent of a McDonald's Big Mac or two slices of pizza, would require forty-five minutes of running, fifty-five minutes of biking, or two hours of walking. Refer to the table on page 19 to learn how many calories you can burn doing various exercises or performing daily chores for a thirty-minute period.

AVERAGE CALORIES BURNED IN VARIOUS PHYSICAL ACTIVITIES

Activity / Calories Burned Per $1/2$ Hour	Activity / Calories Burned Per $1/2$ Hour
Aerobics	**Mowing the Lawn /** 150
Low Impact / 205	**Pushing a Child in a Stroller /** 90
High Impact / 240	**Running**
Basketball / 300	*5 miles per hour /* 290
Biking	*6 miles per hour /* 345
Leisurely / 135	**Stretching /** 135
Spinning / 240	**Swimming** (Moderate pace) / 210
Bowling / 105	**Tennis** (Singles) / 210
Boxing (Punching bag) / 200	**Walking**
Carrying an Infant / 125	*3 miles per hour /* 150
Dancing / 200	*4 miles per hour /* 175
Gardening / 185	**Weight Lifting** (Vigorous) / 205
Golfing (Carrying clubs) / 200	**Yoga /** 140

Although calorie restriction may help the pounds come off initially, exercise is necessary for maintaining weight loss and preventing your body from "plateauing," which occurs when weight loss levels off and stops despite continued efforts to reduce. Usually, hitting a weight plateau indicates that an additional change needs to be made in order to jump-start weight loss once again, and exercise is an effective way to do this. You should commit yourself to a structured exercise plan to ensure that you burn calories regularly. Ideally, this plan will incorporate cardiovascular exercise, strength training, and stretching. This way, you will be burning calories while simultaneously building muscle and improving your flexibility.

Exercise should be moderate first, especially if your lifestyle has been mostly sedentary up to this point. Begin to include forms of light physical activity, such as walking and taking the stairs, in your daily routine before starting a more intense workout regimen. Studies have shown that walking on a regular basis not only increases the number of calories your body burns, but also lowers your risk of heart disease, lowers blood pressure, and protects against falling and bone fractures in older people. Stick to exercises that you enjoy so that you stay motivated, but strive for a balanced, well-rounded program. In addition, you should always consult your physician before beginning any exercise plan, particularly if you're unsure of what your body can handle. (For more exercise tips and guidelines, see page 194 of Chapter 20.)

CONCLUSION

Exercise may be your key to weight loss, and, fortunately, your exercise habits are within your power to control and change. The bottom line is this: If you exercise, you burn calories, and if you burn more calories than you consume, you will most likely lose weight. Start by making small changes in your activity level, and increase the intensity or duration of your exercise as your level of fitness permits.

On the other hand, insufficient exercise may be just one of several factors that are keeping you from shedding pounds. If you exercise and are still unable to lose weight, be sure to explore the other chapters in this book, each of which examines a specific lifestyle issue, health problem, or biochemical factor that may be affecting your efforts to reduce. Once you have identified the contributing factors, turn to Chapter 20, "Putting It All Together," which will help you create an integrated weight-loss program that is suited to your needs.

3

Insufficient Fiber Intake

I t's no secret that we live in an age of processed food. Every day, millions of Americans choose prepackaged or fast food over whole, natural foods to save time, money, and energy. It's much easier to unwrap, warm up, or pick up food from a drive-through window than it is to shop for, wash, chop, and cook fresh foods. The result is a lack of nutrients and, as the title of this chapter suggests, too little fiber in our diets.

Although optimal fiber intake is between 30 and 50 grams per day, and the basic requirement recommended by the American Dietetic Association (ADA) is only 25 to 30 grams per day, most people do not get even half of this amount. Most Americans consume approximately 15 grams of fiber on a daily basis, a fact that has only added to national health concerns. Particularly when combined with a high-calorie diet, low fiber intake can be the root cause of weight gain.

WHAT IS FIBER?

Fiber, also referred to as "roughage" or "bulk," is a complex carbohydrate found in fruits, vegetables, whole grains, nuts, and legumes. Fiber does not contain any calories, so it does not cause weight gain, and it is not digested or absorbed by the body. Rather, fiber aids the digestive and absorption processes by moving through the gastrointestinal tract and speeding up the body's removal of waste material.

Fiber is either soluble or insoluble. *Soluble fiber* simultaneously absorbs water and slows the absorption of fat, sugar, and cholesterol in the stomach and intestines. This works to regulate blood sugar levels, lower cholesterol and blood pressure, and promote the growth of good bacteria. Pectins, gums, and mucilages, which are gel-forming fibers found in many fruits and vegetables, fall into the soluble fiber category. *Insoluble fiber* plays a slightly different role, moving through the digestive tract to sweep out the intestines, eliminate waste, and improve bowel regularity. The cellulose, hemicellulose, and lignins that are contained in nuts, whole grains, and many vegetables are all insoluble fibers.

To simplify, soluble fiber is an absorber, and insoluble fiber is a cleanser. The overall function of fiber is to enhance digestion and detoxify your body, and this has a positive effect on weight loss.

WHAT ARE THE SYMPTOMS OF INSUFFICIENT FIBER INTAKE?

If you do not eat fruits, vegetables, and whole grains regularly, you probably aren't getting the fiber needed to enhance digestive health and general well-being. The symptoms of insufficient fiber intake can range from mild abdominal discomfort to diverticulitis, which is inflammation of the intestinal wall. Here are some other indicators that you need to consume more fiber-rich foods:

- Abdominal pain or stomach cramps
- Constipation
- Diet-related nausea
- Excess flatulence
- Frequent hunger
- Hemorrhoids
- Irregular, infrequent, or painful bowel movements

- Irritable bowel syndrome (IBS)
- Loss of appetite
- Overeating
- Proneness to gallstones
- Tiredness or weakness
- Upset stomach
- Varicose veins

There are other negative effects of insufficient fiber consumption that often go unfelt, unseen, and, therefore, undetected. Diabetes, hypertension, high cholesterol, and even colon cancer can stem from a diet lacking in fiber. If you experience one or more of the symptoms listed above, insufficient fiber intake may be contributing to your inability to lose weight.

HOW DOES INSUFFICIENT FIBER CONTRIBUTE TO WEIGHT GAIN?

It may come as a surprise that you can put on weight by *not* eating something, but this is the case when it comes to fiber. First of all, because fiber does not contain any calories, foods that are rich in it are generally less fattening and less calorically dense. For example, a large salad filled with leafy greens has fewer calories than even a single slice of pizza. Second, fiber fills you up more quickly and stays in your system longer, effectively curbing your appetite. This, of course, will prevent you from overeating—which is why starting your meal with a salad of greens and vegetables is never a bad idea.

Fiber also balances your insulin levels, which prevents the storage of extra fat and wards off tiredness as well as sugar cravings. (To learn more about insulin and weight gain, see Chapter 16.) Your body produces more insulin when it does not get enough fiber, and this usually results in eating foods with high sugar content. Sugary foods are mostly empty in terms of nutrients and, therefore, they do not fill you up. You remain hungry, you eat more, and the vicious cycle continues as you put on additional pounds.

HOW DO YOU DETERMINE IF YOU GET ENOUGH FIBER?

Even if none of the symptoms listed on page 22 apply to you, it's still possible that your fiber intake is inadequate. Many people who are in the habit of eating fast food lunches and microwaveable dinners do not get the basic fiber requirement recommended by the ADA. Those who follow high-protein, low-carb diets also often neglect to eat enough fiber, since meat and dairy products contain an insignificant amount, if any. Moreover, commonly consumed foods like white bread, rice, pasta, sugary cereals, cookies, cakes, and fruit juice are also low in fiber, despite their high carbohydrate content.

If you're concerned that your fiber intake is too low, start paying attention to the nutrition labels on the foods you are buying and eating. As with other important nutrients, the amount of dietary fiber a food contains is always provided on the package label. If the listed amount is 5 grams or more per serving, the food can be considered fiber-rich. A "good" source of fiber contains anywhere from 2.5 to 4.9 grams per serving. To put this in perspective, a medium-sized apple contains approximately 4 grams of fiber, a sweet potato has about 6 grams, and a single cup of cooked beans or lentils can contain 15 grams. Keep track of how much fiber you are consuming on a daily basis, and aim for at least 30 grams per day.

WHAT CAN YOU DO TO LOSE WEIGHT?

If you think fiber insufficiency is the reason behind your inability to lose weight, there are several ways you can incorporate more fiber into your diet. A common misconception about fiber is that eating salad is the only way to ensure you're getting enough. Although green, leafy vegetables are certainly healthy and abundant in fiber, there are other foods you can add to your diet that will allow you to get the recommended 30 grams without having to sacrifice your personal preferences. The following lists present a sampling of foods that contain healthy amounts of soluble and insoluble fiber. Ideally, your diet should be rich in items from both lists so that you get both types of healthful fiber.

Food Sources of Soluble Fiber

- Apples
- Apricots
- Bananas
- Barley
- Beans (kidney, lima, navy, pinto)
- Broccoli
- Cabbage
- Chickpeas
- Flaxseed
- Grapefruit
- Nuts
- Oat bran
- Okra
- Oranges
- Pears
- Prunes
- Psyllium
- Split peas
- Sweet potatoes

Food Sources of Insoluble Fiber

- Bananas
- Beans
- Broccoli
- Brown rice
- Brussels sprouts
- Cauliflower
- Celery
- Corn
- Crackers
- Grains
- High-fiber cereal
- Lentils
- Nuts
- Pasta

- Potatoes (with skin)
- Prunes
- Spinach

- Wheat bran (unprocessed)
- Whole wheat bread

Simply replacing refined grains with whole grains, and adding servings of fruits or vegetables to your meals will increase your fiber consumption. Remember to step up your fiber intake gradually (and drink plenty of water) so that you don't experience any irritating or uncomfortable side effects. Too much fiber often causes bloating, constipation, cramping, and indigestion. It may take a few weeks for your digestive system to fully adjust to a fiber increase.

If you continue to experience the symptoms of a fiber deficiency even after making adjustments to your diet, you may want to consider taking a fiber supplement. There are several popular brands geared to different health goals, including weight management, nutrition, immunity, and bowel regularity. Just be sure to check the amount of carbohydrates and sugar the supplement contains before purchasing, as manufacturers often add these ingredients to appeal to consumers. Drinking enough water is especially important when taking fiber supplements, so stay hydrated for optimal results.

CONCLUSION

You will be well on your way to controlling your weight if you begin to include fruits, vegetables, grains, and nuts in your meals and snacks. Try to eat whole, fresh foods whenever possible, and read the ingredients and nutrition labels before purchasing anything packaged and processed. A balanced, healthy diet is important regardless of whether or not you are overweight.

On the other hand, insufficient fiber may be just one of several factors that are keeping you from shedding pounds. If you eat fiber and are still unable to lose weight, be sure to explore the other chapters in this book, each of which examines a specific lifestyle issue, health problem, or biochemical factor that may be affecting your efforts to reduce. Once you have identified the contributing factors, turn to Chapter 20, "Putting It All Together," which will help you create an integrated weight-loss program that is suited to your needs.

4

Food Addiction

If you're like most people, you've been guilty of overeating at some point in your life. It may have been a response to stress, depression, or boredom; the lure of a delicious meal on some holiday; or the simple result of not having eaten enough during the day, leading to an evening binge. Your overindulgence may also have been caused by a craving for a particular sugary, salty, or fattening food, which made it difficult to stop eating once you started. These are common scenarios—overeating and food cravings are not restricted to those who suffer from weight gain. When these cravings become constant, uncontrollable, and an accepted way of life, however, the problem is more serious than the simple love of food or a lack of willpower. Rather, your urge to eat and the resulting pounds may be caused by an addiction to food that is as physiological as it is mental.

WHAT IS FOOD ADDICTION?

Food addiction, also called *compulsive overeating,* is a clinical disorder characterized by the excessive craving and overconsumption of food. Food addicts eat for pleasure, not out of a physical need for calories, and are preoccupied with thoughts of the foods they crave most intensely. For many years, it was widely assumed that food addiction stemmed solely from an emotional issue, and that a food addict's dependency was purely psychological. Recently, however, scientists have found that certain commonly eaten foods—chocolate, cheese, and bread, to name a few—can be *physically* addictive and affect the brain's chemical balance by stimulating its pleasure center.

When chocolate or some other sugar-laden food is eaten, it acts like an opiate in the brain, giving you a "high" much like caffeine, morphine, marijuana, and amphetamines. This also happens when you eat refined carbohydrates like white flour as well as most dairy products. These substances alter the brain's chemistry, elevating levels of dopamine and serotonin, which are the "feel good" neurotransmitters that regulate mood and appetite. (To read more about neurotransmitters, see Chapter 18.) By linking the eating behavior with pleasurable feelings, your brain makes you want to repeat that behavior. In other words, your brain triggers cravings for the very foods that caused a chemical imbalance in the first place. Eating more allows you to experience another "high," but, as with drugs and alcohol, the high is temporary and only leaves you wanting more. People with diabetes, food intolerances, and unidentified food allergies may get a similar "high" from the foods to which they have the greatest sensitivity. (See Chapter 8 for more on food allergies.) These individuals, therefore, crave and risk becoming addicted to foods that will potentially harm them.

Researchers have also made a connection between the physical addictiveness of particular foods and human biology. Early humans did not have year-round access to fruits and other foods rich in sugar and carbohydrates, so when the foods were available, people were forced to consume them in significant amounts as a means of storing energy. Because survival was dependent on the overconsumption of these foods, it was important that they be both physically addicting and enjoyable to eat. The pleasurable effect of eating these foods functioned as a way of reinforcing a behavior upon which the existence of human beings was hinged.

Unfortunately, overindulging in sugar and carbs is no longer a basic necessity, but a widespread health problem made worse by the fact that so much of the food that is sold, bought, and eaten today contains addictive ingredients. The more you eat, the more you need to appease your appetite, enhance your mood, and boost your energy. In addition, you may experience symptoms of withdrawal if your consumption of certain foods suddenly stops. What was once a means of survival has developed into not only an accepted bad habit, but a growing—and often unrecognized—addiction.

WHAT ARE THE SYMPTOMS OF FOOD ADDICTION?

Although some food addicts may demonstrate a variety of compulsive behaviors, their reliance on food for pleasure and satisfaction is the most overpowering. Some of the symptoms of food addiction are:

- Compulsively overeating, despite not being physically hungry
- Craving certain kinds of food
- Eating rapidly
- Eating to the point of physical sickness
- Feeling guilty or anxious while or after eating
- Frequent stress brought on by worrying about food or eating behaviors
- Hoarding or hiding food
- Knowingly eating foods that may be harmful
- Low self-esteem
- Obsessively craving and thinking about food
- Turning to food to relieve stress or deal with unpleasant emotions
- Viewing food as harmful or something to be avoided

Aside from weight gain, food addicts may experience a number of physical symptoms, many of which are associated with other forms of addiction. These include, but are not limited to, the following:

- Depression
- Headaches
- Insomnia
- Irritability
- Mood changes
- Sluggishness (due to overeating)
- Stomach cramps or nausea

Food addicts can also exhibit signs of physical and emotional withdrawal. Some may avoid social activities, and instead spend their time dealing with feelings of guilt and shame caused by overeating. In extreme cases of food addiction, people can experience tremors as a result of physical withdrawal. If several of these symptoms sound familiar to you, a food addiction may be contributing to your weight-loss problems.

HOW DOES FOOD ADDICTION CONTRIBUTE TO WEIGHT GAIN?

It goes without saying that overeating and binging on foods high in fats, sugar, and refined carbohydrates will cause you to put on pounds. But it's

The Addictive Power of Fructose

Sugar, chocolate, bread—these are all foods that people tend to crave and overeat. As you've learned in this chapter, this is true not just because we find these foods delicious, but also because they affect the brain's chemical balance, giving us a high, much like drugs. According to a study at the University of California, perhaps the worst of these foods is sugar, and perhaps the worst type of sugar is fructose.

When eaten in excess, *all sugar* is unhealthy. It makes the brain think it's hungry, it causes sugar cravings, and it can lead to insulin resistance. Of course, it's also high in calories and causes weight gain. But researchers have found that, although fructose and other sugars have the same amount of calories, fructose generates even greater insulin resistance than products like table sugar because it is absorbed by the body more quickly. This, in turn, makes fructose even more likely to cause increased appetite and cravings, and, over time, to create more serious health problems, such as diabetes. (For more information on insulin resistance, see Chapter 16.) Some researchers also believe that fructose is as harmful as alcohol in that it causes fat storage in the liver, which can lead to fatty liver disease. It also appears to elevate levels of LDL ("bad") cholesterol and triglycerides. Medical trials also suggest that consuming high levels of fructose can lead to kidney stone formation, hypertension, and even gout.

Fructose is found naturally in fruits and vegetables such as corn. This produce is fine because it pairs the sugar with satisfying fiber and other health-promoting nutrients. But over the past century, Americans have increased their consumption of fructose from 15 grams per day to more than 75 grams a day as fructose has become a popular ingredient in processed foods. Now, inexpensive high-fructose corn syrup has become a standard component of soft drinks, breads, breakfast bars, cereals, yogurts, and other commercial products. The bottom line is that to lose weight, you have to cut down on sugar, and to avoid serious health problems and beat food addictions, you and your family should especially avoid processed foods that contain the sugar known as fructose.

what happens inside your body when you consume such substances that explains why weight gain is the outcome of food addiction.

As you may recall from Chapter 1, your body's hunger and fullness levels are determined by two hormones, *ghrelin* and *leptin*. Ghrelin stimulates your appetite while leptin suppresses it, sending signals to your brain to let you know you're full. Eating nutritious foods on a regular schedule each day balances the production of these two important substances. Not surprisingly, the kinds of foods that increase the body's secretion of ghrelin are also the most physically addictive. Furthermore, scientists have discovered that overweight and obese people have higher levels of ghrelin than do thinner individuals, which means that they are hungrier more often. This paints a grim picture for those people who are overweight and *also* addicted to food. Whereas people of normal weight may need only a bite or two of cake to be satisfied, overweight and obese people may need a generous slice, and overweight food addicts may need the entire cake, both to satisfy their appetite and get a "high." Their addiction to the food overrides their body's actual needs until it becomes a physiological dependency that traps them in an ongoing cycle—one that puts them on the fast-track to weight gain and related problems such as heart disease.

HOW DO YOU DETERMINE IF YOU HAVE A FOOD ADDICTION?

If you are unsure whether your eating behaviors are symptoms of food addiction or simply bad habits, there are several factors you should consider. Start by looking at the foods you eat most frequently. Although it is difficult to pin down the "typical" diet of a food addict, most binge on foods high in fat, salt, and sugar, or constantly graze on them throughout the day. Next, assess *how* you eat. This can be done by asking yourself the following questions:

- Do you eat when you are truly hungry, or because you are anxious, sad, or stressed?

- Do you find it difficult to stop eating once you start, no matter how full you are?

- Do you frequently worry about food and your eating habits?

- Do you eat secretly?

- Do you eat differently in private than in front of others?

- Do you obsessively count calories or severely restrict your food intake?

- Do you hoard or hide food?

- Do you feel guilty or ashamed after overeating, and then spend hours dwelling on it?

- Do your eating behaviors interfere with your daily activities, work, or social relationships?

If you cannot lose weight and answered "yes" to any of the questions above, a food addiction may be affecting your weight-loss efforts. It is important to note, however, that food addicts are not necessarily over-weight. In more extreme cases, people may counteract binges through vomiting, laxatives, or excessive exercise in an attempt to burn off calo-ries. Those who use these methods may be of normal weight, and, if their disorder is particularly severe, they may even be underweight. Still, weight gain is one of the most common and noticeable physical symp-toms of food addiction. So if you're concerned that your eating behaviors are contributing to your weight problem, you should seek the advice of a medical professional who is trained in metabolic or bariatric medicine. (See the "Resources" section for information on how to find health prac-titioners in your area.)

WHAT CAN YOU DO TO LOSE WEIGHT?

There is no "cure" for an addiction to food anymore than there is for addictions to other substances. Professional counseling and support groups will make the road to recovery easier, but full treatment depends largely on lifestyle change. Food addicts need to identify and replace the unhealthy foods they crave with ones rich in nutrients and fiber. (For a list of good food sources of fiber, see Chapter 3.) Here are some other ways you can control and treat food addiction:

- Avoid situations or foods that will stimulate cravings.

- Drink eight glasses (or 64 ounces) of water every day. (If you have heart or kidney problems, you should speak to your doctor about appropri-ate water consumption.)

- Eat three reasonable, nutritious meals each day on a regular schedule, beginning with a balanced breakfast in the morning. If your schedule permits, eating five smaller meals every day may be even more advan-tageous for weight management.

- Engage in enjoyable, relaxing activities (meditation, yoga, reading, etc.) that distract you from your food cravings.

- Exercise as your level of physical fitness allows, gradually increasing intensity and duration. (See Chapter 2 for more about exercise.)

By introducing these smaller changes into your life, you will be able to get better control of your eating behaviors, compulsions, and appetite. A lifestyle that incorporates the healthy habits listed above will also go a long way in promoting weight loss.

CONCLUSION

Because cutting food out of your life entirely is not an option, overcoming food addiction is a difficult struggle. But by recognizing the problem and working towards healthier habits, you can break the addiction cycle and shed extra pounds.

Even if you do suffer from an addiction to food, there may be other factors that are preventing you from losing weight. If you get treatment for your addiction and continue to gain weight, be sure to explore the other chapters in this book. Each examines a specific lifestyle issue, health problem, or biochemical factor that may have a negative impact on your efforts to reduce. Once you have identified the contributing factors, turn to Chapter 20, "Putting It All Together," which will help you create an integrated weight-loss program that is suited to your needs.

5

Sleep Deprivation

I t's 6:00 AM, and your alarm is buzzing. But instead of going to the gym as you intended, you hit the "Snooze" button and roll over to get some extra shuteye before work. You end up dragging yourself out of bed to get to the office on time, and much of the day is spent making trips to the coffee machine or munching on sugary snacks to keep yourself alert. Later, you decide to skip the gym (who wants to exercise after a long day?), and because you simply don't have the energy to cook dinner, you pick up a pizza on your way home. Your evening consists of lounging on the couch in front of the TV or catching up on the work you couldn't seem to focus on during the day—all while snacking, of course. So much for getting to bed early. By midnight, you're completely drained, but you lie awake thinking about everything you neglected to do that day. You have just barely started to doze when the sun comes up, and you begin the same old routine once again, just as exhausted as you were the day before.

Sound familiar? If so, you aren't alone. An approximated 60 million Americans suffer from some kind of sleep loss due to poor diet, lack of exercise, excessive caffeine intake, hectic schedules, or life's usual stresses. Unfortunately, rather than treat their disrupted sleep patterns as a health issue, many people make the mistake of believing they can get by on little—if any—sleep. But this thinking seriously impacts their health. Hypertension, insulin resistance, and heart disease have all been linked to sleep deprivation, and severe cases of the condition can produce symptoms typically associated with the beginning stages of psychosis, including hallucinations and tremors. Moreover, sleeplessness can sabotage your weight-reduction efforts, since metabolism and appetite are affected by how much you sleep each night. Consequently, millions of sleep-deprived people are struggling to shed pounds and can't figure out what is preventing them from doing so.

WHAT IS SLEEP DEPRIVATION?

Sleep deprivation can generally be defined as a lack of sleep over an extended period of time, causing physical or psychiatric symptoms and affecting the routine performance of tasks. Sleep deprivation ranges from partial or restless sleep to chronic insomnia—sleeplessness that lasts for longer than three weeks. When you don't get an adequate amount of sleep, your body does not have the time it needs to repair itself, which makes you more susceptible to illness, injury, stress, mood swings, and general fatigue—and these are only minor effects when compared to the medical issues mentioned earlier. Most doctors estimate that the average adult needs between seven and nine hours of sleep each night to detoxify the body, conserve energy, and maintain proper immune, neurological, and cognitive function, but a number of factors can hinder you from getting the recommended amount. Some of the underlying reasons for sleep deprivation are:

- A diet that includes excessive caffeine, alcohol, chocolate, spicy foods, additives, or, for people who are gluten sensitive, wheat products.

- Food allergies. (See Chapter 8.)

- Hormonal imbalances, including elevated cortisol, low estrogen (women), low growth hormone, low melatonin, low progesterone (women), low testosterone (men), or thyroid dysfunction. (See Chapters 10, 14, and 17 for more information about hormonal imbalances.)

- Insufficient exercise.

- Medical conditions such as anxiety disorder, asthma, chronic pain, depression, gallbladder disease, hiatal hernia/reflux esophagitis, nasal and sinus problems, and urinary disorders.

- Medications, including asthma, blood pressure, and sleep disorder medications, as well as synthetic progestins.

- Neurotransmitter dysfunction. (See Chapter 18.)

- Nutritional deficiencies in copper, iron, magnesium, niacin, tryptophan, vitamin B_6, etc.

- A poor sleeping environment, such as one that includes bright lights or excessive noise.

- Shift work.

- Sleep disorders, particularly sleep apnea.

- Stress.

- Weight-loss supplements.

Whether one of these factors is causing irregular sleep patterns or complete sleep loss, sleeping less than seven hours a night on a consistent basis disturbs your internal balance, which has consequences for your general well-being.

WHAT ARE THE SYMPTOMS OF SLEEP DEPRIVATION?

Regardless of whether you average six hours of sleep each night or barely two, you undoubtedly feel the effects of sleep deprivation. In addition to general sleepiness (and weight gain), you may experience one or more of the following symptoms:

- Changes in appetite
- Depression
- Fatigue
- Food cravings
- Headaches
- Inability to concentrate
- Increased anxiety or stress

- Irritability
- Low productivity
- Memory lapse or loss
- Mood fluctuations
- Muscle aches
- Nystagmus (eye twitch)
- Slow reaction time

If you have experienced several of these symptoms, then sleep deprivation may be contributing to your weight-loss problem.

HOW DOES SLEEP DEPRIVATION CONTRIBUTE TO WEIGHT GAIN?

If the connection between lack of sleep and weight gain is not immediately obvious, consider how your eating habits change when you feel like you're running on empty. You may find that you're quicker to reach for a doughnut, cookie, or candy bar due to increased hunger and sugar cravings. You may also turn to high-calorie caffeinated beverages in an effort to improve your energy level and get through the day without crashing. If this is the case, you're not alone. Sleep deprivation significantly impacts your appetite and how you metabolize the foods you eat.

The Melatonin Connection

How well you sleep is largely determined by the level of certain hormones in your body, including ACTH, cortisol, FSH, LH, prolactin, TSH, and, perhaps most important of all, melatonin. Insomnia is often attributed to low levels of melatonin, which is the hormone that sets your body's twenty-four-hour cycle and influences your sleep habits, mood, immunity, and response to stress. When the sun goes down, the brain's pineal gland is stimulated to produce melatonin and then release it into the bloodstream, which causes you to feel drowsy. However, there are several factors that can inhibit this process, including:

- Alcohol
- Alpha adrenergic blockers
- Aspirin
- Beta blockers
- Caffeine
- Calcium channel blockers
- Electromagnetic fields (computer, TV, and other electronic devices)
- Excessive exposure to light
- Exercising less than three hours before bedtime
- Ibuprofen and other non-steroidal anti-inflammatory drugs
- Steroids
- Tobacco
- Tranquilizers

Since melatonin is also instrumental in growth hormone production, cancer prevention, and bone formation, it is important to produce a sufficient amount. If you think one or more of the factors above may be connected to your sleep deficit, you can increase your melatonin naturally by eating foods such as bananas, cherries, corn, oats, rice, and onions. These foods contain a small amount of melatonin, as do foods rich in B vitamins (whole grains, legumes, leafy vegetables) and tryptophan (chicken, beef, dairy products, and nuts). You can also contact a laboratory that will test your saliva to determine if your melatonin level is too low. (See page 207 of "Resources" for a list of diagnostic laboratories.)

You may recall from Chapter 1 that two hormones are responsible for appetite regulation. *Ghrelin* stimulates feelings of hunger, while *leptin* sends signals to your brain to let you know you're full. Normally, these hormones function as a system of checks and balances, but a sleep deficit upsets this system. The sleep-deprived body produces more ghrelin and less leptin, and this combination makes for a greater appetite that is difficult to satisfy. In other words, insufficient sleep leads to overeating, which, of course, promotes weight gain.

Several medical studies have found that sleep loss may trigger cravings for foods rich in carbohydrates and sugars, as they provide short bursts of energy. The same studies have also produced evidence that sleep deprivation interferes with your body's ability to metabolize these foods. When carbohydrates are processed more slowly, more of the food is stored as fat, leading to yet more weight gain. Moreover, the high intake of carbs causes a spike in blood sugar, which increases your body's insulin levels as well as your tolerance for sugar. (See Chapter 16 to learn more about insulin resistance and weight-loss problems.) Even a few nights of sleeplessness can make you more insulin resistant and put you on the path to extra pounds.

HOW DO YOU DETERMINE IF YOU ARE SLEEP DEPRIVED?

Sleeping for a solid eight hours is a novelty rather than the norm for most people. In effect, many do not realize they are sleep deprived, and end up ignoring their symptoms or attributing them to some other cause. Although the amount of sleep needed to function at an optimal level varies from person to person, most doctors consider less than six to seven hours of sleep to be inadequate, and sleeping less than this amount on a consistent basis is sleep deprivation.

To determine if you suffer from a sleep deficit, start paying attention to how you feel during the day. If you frequently feel the urge to take a nap, require several cups of coffee just make it to lunchtime, or have difficulty staying awake when you're doing seated activities such as desk work, watching TV, or reading, you are probably not sleeping enough. In addition, if you find yourself snapping at others or stuck in a habitual bad mood, you should evaluate the reasons behind your irritability. A lack of sleep can make you emotionally unstable, and moodiness is a key indicator.

You may want to consider starting a sleep journal to keep track of the total amount you sleep each night, recording the times you go to bed and wake up in the morning. This journal can also be used to write about the quality of your sleep, including the occasions when you wake up several times during the night, get up for a midnight snack, or lay awake stressing about various problems. After a couple weeks of writing about your sleeping issues, you may notice patterns that will help you identify the factors that are causing sleeplessness so you can deal with them appropriately. A journal may tell you whether you need to eat a more satisfying snack at night, resolve a problem that is troubling you, or seek treatment for a more serious disorder or illness.

WHAT CAN YOU DO TO LOSE WEIGHT?

There are several ways you can get a good night's sleep without the aid of medications. Here are some suggestions for strengthening your sleep patterns naturally:

- Regularize your sleeping schedule by going to bed at the same time every night and arising at the same time every morning. Don't deviate too far from this schedule on weekends, and try to avoid prolonged daytime naps.

- Make your bed a "sleep-only zone"—avoid doing work or watching TV there. This way, you'll associate it *only* with slumber and nod off more quickly and easily, especially if you keep your bedroom cool, dark, and quiet.

- Kick the caffeine and sugar habits. You may think high-sugar snacks and caffeinated beverages are the only things that are keeping you going, but they're also keeping you up at night. Other unhealthy habits like excessive drinking and smoking can also disturb your sleep patterns, which is another reason you should put an end to these behaviors.

- Don't go to bed hungry. Have a small, healthy snack a couple of hours before bedtime to stabilize your blood sugar and keep you satisfied all night. Complex carbohydrates and low-fat proteins will accomplish this, so try eating a small bowl of whole grain cereal, a banana with eight to ten almonds, or half of a turkey sandwich on whole wheat bread, and wash it down with a cup of hot herbal tea. Other foods that promote sleep are lemons, mulberries, mushrooms, and vegetables high in chlorophyll such as spinach, green olives, asparagus, and broccoli.

- Fit exercise into your day a few times a week. This will help you deal with any stress that may keep you tossing and turning all night long, as well as make your sleep deeper, longer, and more restful. Keep in mind, however, that a vigorous exercise session right before bed will prevent sleep, so if you can find time to work out only in the evening, complete your routine as early as possible and stick to activities that are of light or moderate intensity.

You'll probably notice a difference in your sleeping patterns when you make these small lifestyle changes. If you still experience difficulty falling asleep, or if you continue to suffer from insomnia, there are nutritional supplements you can take to improve your sleep quality. The substances listed in the table below can be effective alternatives to sleeping pills and prescription sleep aids.

SUPPLEMENTS TO TREAT INSOMNIA

Supplement	Dosage	Considerations
Astragalus	500 mg once a day.	Should not be used by anyone who has a gum allergy, has had an organ transplant, or suffers from an autoimmune disease such as rheumatoid arthritis (RA), multiple sclerosis (MS), or lupus. Astragalus may raise blood sugar and blood pressure. Usually used in combination with other herbs.
Chamomile	Make into a tea and drink three to four times daily, or take 100 mg in capsule form once a day.	As it makes users drowsy, do not drink alcohol or other sedatives after consuming chamomile. In addition, chamomile should not be taken with anti-coagulants or by anyone who has difficulty clotting blood. Do not take if you are allergic to ragweed or related plants.
5-HTP (5-hydroxy-tryptophan)	25 to 150 mg twice a day.*	Do not take 5-HTP if you are taking an SSRI, MAO inhibitor, or other antidepressant.
GABA (Gamma-aminobutyric acid)	• If you weigh less than 125 pounds, take 375 mg three times a day. • If you weigh more than 125 pounds, take 750 mg three times a day.	GABA may cause a tingling sensation in the face and slight shortness of breath; this should last for only a few minutes. GABA may make you drowsy, so take it in the evening. Do not take GABA if you have kidney or liver disease.

Hop strobile (hops)	50 mg once a day.	Do not take with sedative medications. People who suffer from depression should not take hops, since it may worsen symptoms. Do not take if you are pregnant or breastfeeding. Stop taking hops at least two weeks before a scheduled surgery. Do not take if you are allergic to hops.
Lemon balm	600 mg once a day.	Do not take if you are pregnant or breastfeeding.
L-theanine	200 to 400 mg twice a day.*	Do not use if you are taking blood pressure medication or stimulant drugs. Women who are pregnant or breast-feeding should avoid use. L-theanine is intended for short-term use only.
Magnesium	400 to 800 mg once a day.*	Consult health-care provider for dosage if you have kidney disease. Discontinue use and see your doctor if you experience abdominal pain. Take a lower dose if it causes diarrhea. Magnesium's citrate, glycinate, gluconate, and lactate forms are more easily absorbed than its oxide form.
Magnolia bark extract (*Magnolia officinalis*)	250 to 750 mg of 1- to 2-percent honokiol and magnolol extract once a day.*	Do not take with sedative medications, as magnolia may cause drowsiness. Magnolia may also induce miscarriages, so women who are pregnant should not use under any circumstances. Do not take if you are breastfeeding or undergoing surgery.
Melatonin	1 to 6 mg once a day, before bedtime.*	For ideal use, take thirty minutes before bedtime while in a dark room. Start by taking 1 mg and increase your dose as needed. People who are pregnant, take prescription steroids, or have depression, mental illness, leukemia, lymphoma, or an autoimmune disease should not take melatonin. Possible side effects include headache, fatigue, and nightmares.
Passion flower	50 mg once a day.	Do not use passion flower if you are pregnant, breastfeeding, or taking an MAO inhibitor to treat depression. Stop taking two weeks before any scheduled surgery. Always avoid high dosages, as they may cause some people to experience an irregular heartbeat, nausea, and dizziness.

*To choose an appropriate dose, see page 199 for information on dosage ranges.

Remember, if you are unsure whether you should be taking a certain supplement, consult a medical professional beforehand. Stop using any supplement if you experience symptoms that concern you.

CONCLUSION

Never underestimate the power of a good night's sleep, particularly when planning a weight-loss program. Although eight hours is ideal, seven is enough to ward off weight gain and enhance your overall health. Dietary modifications, regular workouts, and a sleep-friendly environment can go a long way when it comes to achieving restful sleep each night, which will, in turn, help you reach a healthier weight.

On the other hand, sleep deprivation may be just one of several factors that are keeping you from shedding pounds. If you take steps to correct the problem and still are unable to lose weight, be sure to explore the other chapters in this book, each of which examines a specific lifestyle issue, health problem, or biochemical factor that may be affecting your efforts to reduce. Once you have identified the contributing factors, turn to Chapter 20, "Putting It All Together," which will help you create an integrated weight-loss program that is suited to your needs.

6

Stress

If you've ever had to meet a tight deadline, pass an important exam, pay a stack of bills, or score a point with only seconds on the clock, then you know what stress feels like. You probably felt tense, yet more focused and alert. Your heart may have pounded more quickly when you looked at the calendar, scoreboard, or pile of papers. In all likelihood, you also experienced a surge of energy as you raced to accomplish the task at hand. These sensations are all part of your body's *stress response*, a "fight or flight" reaction that functions to help you meet and overcome challenges. It is the reason why you can successfully get through a presentation, score the winning goal, stay up late to finish work, and fight to protect yourself in life-threatening situations. Although the word is often used negatively, stress is a necessary—and perhaps beneficial—part of life; stress keeps you sharp and focused, it forces you to be productive, and it can even save your life.

Still, there is a fine line between healthy and unhealthy stress, or *distress*. Long-term stress can pose a serious hazard to your health, increasing your risk of heart attack, stroke, digestive problems, autoimmune diseases, and depression. In addition, the stress hormones released to give you stamina and put you in "survival mode" also affect metabolism, body fat storage, blood sugar, and food cravings, which can lead to added pounds. But by finding out how stress works in your body, you can learn how to cope in a healthy way and ward off the weight gain it can cause.

WHAT IS STRESS?

Stress is your body's physical, mental, and emotional response to pressure from both external factors, such as job demands and busy schedules, and internal factors, like negativity and perfectionism. Your body is biologically hardwired to protect itself against various *stressors,* and it is able to do so because two hormones—chemical "messengers" in the body that regulate its activities—work together to keep you cheerful, energetic, and clear-headed. These hormones, manufactured in the adrenal glands, are *cortisol,* the so-called "stress hormone," and *dehydroepiandrosterone (DHEA),* which is mainly responsible for making sure your body has sufficient amounts of hormones when it needs them. In periods of non-stress, cortisol and DHEA both play a role in brain function, mood regulation, immunity, and weight control. But when you are stressed, an adequate amount of DHEA allows your body to increase its production of cortisol, which gives you more energy, better immunity, and higher tolerance for pain.

However, problems arise when you experience a significant amount of stress for an extended length of time, or *chronic stress.* Elevated cortisol is beneficial in the short-term—it activates the metabolism of fats and carbohydrates for quick energy and keeps your blood sugar level stable. But

What Is Adrenal Fatigue?

Although you may not be familiar with it, adrenal fatigue is not uncommon. It is the "state of emergency" for the adrenal glands, and it affects those who are regularly exposed to high-stress situations—caregivers, health-care providers, and competitive athletes, for instance— and those who have experienced traumas, such as victims of crimes and car accidents. Basically, adrenal fatigue occurs when your glands can no longer keep up with the level of stress you are experiencing, and they begin to produce only enough cortisol and DHEA to keep you alive rather than protect and sustain your body. There are numerous symptoms of adrenal fatigue, but the disorder often goes undetected by doctors, instead dismissed as stress or extreme fatigue. In addition to feeling generally rundown, symptoms of adrenal fatigue include:

- Apathy, or loss of interest in activities once enjoyed
- Chronic fatigue
- Cravings for foods high in fat, salt, and sugar
- Decreased sex drive
- Development of allergies with severe reactions, including rashes and dermatitis
- Frequent hyperventilation (abnormally fast or deep breathing)

over time, high amounts of cortisol can lead to sleep disturbances, increased blood pressure and cholesterol, irritability, sugar cravings, insulin resistance, and an energy deficit, among other health issues. On the other hand, prolonged stress ultimately results in *decreased* DHEA, since your body cannot produce enough to keep up with the level of stress you're experiencing. This results in an overall hormonal imbalance and generates feelings of depression. The combination of low DHEA and high cortisol increases your body's fat storage, stimulates appetite, slows metabolism, and decreases muscle mass. In more severe cases of chronic stress, the overproduction of your stress hormone can result in *adrenal fatigue*, which is essentially a state of "burnout" for your adrenal glands. Your glands then become unable to make enough cortisol, resulting in a cortisol deficiency and intensified stress symptoms that pose a greater risk to your health. (To learn more about adrenal fatigue, see the inset on pages 46 to 47.)

- Hypoglycemia (low blood sugar), usually stress-induced

- Inability to concentrate

- Increased susceptibility to illness and infection with slow recovery

- Irregular bowel movements

- Loss of motivation, initiative, and stamina

- Nervousness, excessive fear, and constant feelings of being overwhelmed

- Poor digestion

- Progressively poorer athletic performance

- Recurring respiratory infections

Along with these side effects, people who suffer from adrenal fatigue also report marital discord, less productivity at work, decreased social activity, and unusual sleep patterns—their most refreshing sleep takes place between 7:00 AM and 9:00 AM. If you are concerned that you have adrenal fatigue, you should consult a physician who specializes in metabolic and anti-aging medicine. Adrenal fatigue is sometimes mistaken for thyroid dysfunction (see Chapter 10), so it's a good idea to have a doctor measure your cortisol level to determine the real cause of your symptoms.

WHAT ARE THE SYMPTOMS OF STRESS?

The effects of stress vary from individual to individual, with the possible symptoms falling into four separate categories: behavioral, cognitive (related to thinking, reasoning, and remembering), emotional, and physical, as shown in the lists below. While it is highly unlikely that all or even most of these symptoms will affect you, keep in mind that experiencing even a few is cause for concern.

Behavioral Symptoms

- Compulsive eating
- Critical attitude
- Difficulty completing tasks
- Disrupted sleep
- Grinding of teeth while sleeping
- Increased alcohol consumption
- Neglecting responsibilities
- Smoking or drug use
- Short temper

Cognitive Symptoms

- Anxious or racing thoughts
- Constant worry
- Forgetfulness
- Inability to make decisions
- Negativity
- Poor judgment
- Trouble thinking clearly or focusing

Emotional Symptoms

- Anger
- Anxiety
- Apathy or boredom
- Depression
- Easily upset
- Feeling overwhelmed and powerless to change things
- Loneliness
- Moodiness

Physical Symptoms

- Aches and pains
- Bowel movement irregularities
- Chest pain
- Decreased interest in sex
- Dizziness
- Fatigue

- Headaches
- Indigestion
- Nausea

- Rapid heartbeat
- Ringing in ears
- Weight gain

If several of these symptoms sound familiar to you, stress may be contributing to your inability to lose weight.

HOW DOES STRESS CONTRIBUTE TO WEIGHT GAIN?

You now know that your reaction to stress is regulated by cortisol, the hormone that triggers your "fight or flight" response, and DHEA, which allows your cortisol level to be elevated in the first place. Although too much DHEA promotes weight gain, cortisol more directly influences how you eat and metabolize food, leading to extra pounds.

First of all, cortisol is an appetite stimulant—it makes you want to eat. In addition, it encourages the release of a certain brain chemical, *neuropeptide Y*, which increases cravings for carbohydrates. This means that you are both eating more frequently and eating foods that affect your blood sugar and fat storage. On top of this, heightened cortisol levels over an extended period of time can alter how your body processes sugar, making you prone to fatigue, mood swings, hyperglycemia (high blood sugar), and insulin resistance.

Doctors and scientists also now know that too much cortisol will slow your metabolism, causing more of the food you eat to be stored as fat. Unfortunately, excessive stress also influences *where* this fat is stored on your body—the abdominal area. Medical research has shown that not only is abdominal weight harder to lose, but it is also the area of greatest concern in terms of health risks. Abdominal fat has been linked to diabetes and heart disease, among other serious medical conditions.

Of course, stress can cause weight gain for reasons that have nothing to do with a hormonal imbalance. Many people tend to deal with stress by eating, which may have more to do with nervous energy than cortisol-induced cravings. The fatigue caused by stress can also affect your food choices; a lack of energy may prompt you to pick up fast food for lunch or dinner instead of preparing a meal. Whether due to hormones or personal coping mechanisms, the connection between stress and weight gain is obvious—a stressful lifestyle is not a healthy lifestyle.

HOW DO YOU DETERMINE IF YOU ARE TOO STRESSED?

More and more, stress is thought of as an unavoidable fact of life. Many people simply accept stress, which can have consequences for both their health and their waistline. If some of the warning signs and symptoms mentioned earlier ring true for you, you should also consider the following questions:

- Do you dread waking up in the morning and find it difficult to get out of bed?

- Are you frequently sick or "under the weather"?

- Are you filled with nervous energy and constant worry?

- Do you avoid interaction with friends, family members, or coworkers?

- Have you experienced severe allergic reactions, breaking out into hives or rashes?

- Do you have muscle aches and pains so often that you now consider it "normal"?

- Do you bicker with or snap at others all the time, even over petty matters?

- Have you taken up smoking or drinking alcohol to deal with your stress load?

- Have you noticed changes in your eating habits, consuming more foods laden with sugar, salt, or fat?

- Do you see a difference in your physical appearance (dark circles under your eyes, hair loss, acne, etc.)?

If your answer to several of these questions is "yes," then it's likely that you are too stressed—and it's impossible to sustain a healthy body (and a healthy weight) when your stress level is in overdrive. There are tests available for measuring the amount of cortisol in your body, which will indicate if you suffer from chronic stress. Although urine and blood samples can be taken to determine this, saliva testing generally yields the most accurate readings. Of course, a lab test is not always necessary, but it can help you and your doctor to choose and implement a plan for relieving your stress symptoms. (For a list of diagnostic laboratories, see page 207 of "Resources.")

WHAT CAN YOU DO TO LOSE WEIGHT?

If you want to put an end to the sluggishness and snacking that's contributing to your weight gain, diminishing your stress is a must. But first you must figure out what's causing you to feel pressured and overwhelmed in the first place. Relationship difficulties, financial responsibilities, and job demands cannot always be eliminated, but by recognizing how you respond to certain stressors, you can learn how to take charge of them. Depending on the cause of your stress, you may find some of the suggestions below helpful:

- Manage your time by making to-do lists or weekly schedules.

- Take up yoga, Tai Chi (a form of Chinese martial arts that incorporates breathing exercises), or meditation to help calm and clear your mind.

- Don't underestimate the importance of a social support network—have coffee or lunch with a friend regularly.

- Engage in activities and hobbies that you enjoy, such as reading, painting, gardening, volunteering, or cooking.

- Exercise to reduce stress naturally and promote weight loss at the same time.

- Limit your caffeine intake—no coffee after 2:00 PM is ideal.

- Eat for wellness. Balanced, nutritious meals will make you feel healthier and more energetic, so that you won't need to reach for sugary snacks or carbs to deal with pressure. A diet rich in fruits, vegetables, lean meats, and fish can also repair the damage that stress does to the body.

In some cases, lifestyle change may not be enough to completely combat stress, particularly if it has led to a more serious condition such as adrenal fatigue. Fortunately, there are nutritional supplements you can take to boost your adrenal function and restore cortisol and DHEA to their normal levels. The table on page 52 highlights the best of these supplements.

Be sure to consult your health-care provider before taking any of the recommended supplements, and remember that dosages may have to be adjusted depending on your individual needs and any health conditions you may have.

SUPPLEMENTS TO NORMALIZE ADRENAL FUNCTION

Supplement	Dosage	Considerations
Ashwaghanda root	500 to 1,000 mg once a day.*	Do not take if you are pregnant. Possible side effects may include nausea, vomiting, and diarrhea.
Bacopa monniera	200 to 250 mg once a day.	Bacopa is intended for short-term use only, and in some cases may cause fatigue, dry mouth, and nausea. Women who are pregnant or breastfeeding should not use.
B-complex vitamins	Choose a B-complex vitamin that provides 10 to 50 mg each of vitamins B_1, B_2, B_3, B_5, and B_6; 200 to 400 mcg of folic acid; and 250 to 500 mcg of B_{12}. Take twice a day.	Speak to your health-care provider before taking if you have diabetes, liver problems, or anemia. B-complex vitamins may interact with certain antibiotics and anti-seizure medications. Whenever taking a B-complex vitamin, always take a multivitamin as well.
Cordyceps	400 mg twice a day.	Do not take if you are pregnant, breastfeeding, or suffering from an autoimmune disease.
Ginseng	500 mg once a day.	Always take with food. Do not take if you are on blood thinners. Use with caution if you have high blood pressure.
Holy basil	500 to 1,000 mg twice a day.*	Do not take if you are pregnant, breast feeding, or use blood thinners, as holy basil can slow blood clotting. In addition, holy basil is intended only for short-term use because the effects of long-term usage are not yet known. Stop using two weeks before any scheduled surgery.
L-carnitine	500 to 1,000 mg once a day.*	Side effects are rare but can include agitation, headache, increased appetite, nausea, skin rashes, and vomiting. Ask your doctor before taking if you have kidney or liver disease.
Licorice root (*Glycyrrhiza glabra*)	600 mg twice a day.	Consult your physician before taking if you have high blood pressure; glaucoma; diabetes; or heart, kidney, or liver disease.
Magnesium	400 to 800 mg once a day.*	Consult health-care provider for dosage if you have kidney disease. Discontinue use and see your doctor if you experience abdominal pain. Take a lower dose if it causes diarrhea. Magnesium's citrate,

		glycinate, gluconate, and lactate forms are more easily absorbed than its oxide form.
Multivitamin, pharmaceutical-grade†	Follow the directions on the bottle.	Make sure to take only a pharmaceutical-grade multivitamin.
Phosphatidyl-serine	300 mg once a day.	Do not take if you are on a blood-thinning medication. Use with caution if you are also taking medication to treat depression, glaucoma, or Alzheimer's disease. Do not take if you are pregnant or breastfeeding. Side effects may include insomnia and stomach upset.
Rhodiola rosea root extract	50 mg twice a day.	Rhodiola is intended for short-term use only, as its long-term effects are not yet known. Do not use if you are pregnant or breastfeeding.
Vitamin C	1,000 mg once a day.	Doses higher than 5,000 mg may cause diarrhea. Mineral ascorbates and Ester-C are buffered forms of vitamin C that lower the chance of diarrhea. Do not take high doses if you are prone to kidney stones or gout.

*To choose an appropriate dose, see page 199 for information on dosage ranges.
† See page 197 for information on pharmaceutical-grade supplements.

CONCLUSION

Stress reduction is key when it comes to maintaining a healthy body, so remember that relaxation is as important to your life—and weight—as proper nutrition, regular exercise, and restful sleep. Once you learn how to alleviate your stress in healthy ways, you will be on your way to easing your weight-loss troubles. Even if a hormonal imbalance is aggravating your stress symptoms, there is a lot you can do to help your body recover and regain your health.

On the other hand, stress may be just one of several factors that are keeping you from shedding pounds. If you take steps to correct this problem and are still unable to lose weight, be sure to explore the other chapters in this book, each of which examines a specific lifestyle issue, health problem, or biochemical factor that may be affecting your efforts to reduce. Once you have identified the contributing factors, turn to Chapter 20, "Putting It All Together," which will help you create an integrated weight-loss program that is suited to your needs.

7

Insufficient Water Intake

Water makes up about 65 percent of the human body, so it's no wonder that it's vital for just about every function your body carries out. It transports nutrients to your organs and tissues, delivers oxygen to your cells, ensures smooth and easy digestion, maintains proper body temperature and pH balance, enhances your metabolism, and gives you energy. In addition, water is one of nature's most effective remedies, relieving constipation, heartburn, migraines, and muscle aches, and working to prevent more serious medical issues like kidney stones, arthritis, and even heart disease.

Water is just as essential for weight loss. While it may be true that drinking water will not alone lead to lost pounds, meeting your daily requirement for this thirst-quenching, calorie-free nutrient will stimulate your metabolism and fill you up—both great ways to drop extra pounds. So before you reach for another soda, juice, or coffee, it makes sense to learn how this simple substance can help you look and feel your best.

WHAT IS INSUFFICIENT WATER INTAKE?

Insufficient water intake occurs when you do not drink enough water for your body to maintain normal functioning. If you're like most people, you drink because you're thirsty, not because you're trying to meet a quota. But since your body loses water naturally over the course of the day, it's important to keep track of your fluid consumption and regularly replenish your body's supply.

It's estimated that the average adult loses 6.3 cups of water a day through urination, and an additional 4 cups (total) through other body functions like bowel movements, perspiration, and breathing. To make up the deficit, doctors recommend drinking 8 to 9 cups of water per day, along with a balanced diet, which usually accounts for 20 percent of your water intake. This amount can vary depending on several factors, including exercise, environment, and health conditions. For instance, people who work out for an hour or more on a regular basis should drink an extra 1.5 to 2.5 cups of water, as should those who live in a warmer climate or at high altitudes. Women who are pregnant or breastfeeding also require more water—approximately 10 and 13 cups, respectively—and people with certain medical issues, like bladder infections or kidney stones, should increase their water consumption as well.

Many people make the mistake of drinking sugary juice, soda, coffee, or tea to avoid the bland, boring taste of water. Worse is the fact that coffee, tea, and sodas are diuretics: Because they encourage frequent urination, they cause you to lose more fluid and can sometimes even dehydrate you. In other words, consumption of certain fluids (though they contain some water) is actually counterproductive when it comes to maintaining sufficient water intake—a good reason for you to stick mainly to H_2O.

WHAT ARE THE SYMPTOMS OF INSUFFICIENT WATER INTAKE?

Because your body is about 65 percent water and your brain is approximately 85 percent water, consuming insufficient amounts of this vital fluid is detrimental to both your physical and mental wellness. Inadequate water intake can lead to mild or moderate dehydration, which may become severe if not treated. The symptoms you may experience include:

- Acne
- Bloating
- Confusion
- Constipation
- Cramps in arms or legs
- Dark yellow urine
- Decreased urination
- Digestive problems, including heartburn and stomachache
- Dizziness
- Dry eyes and skin
- Dry mouth
- Extreme thirst
- Fatigue
- Flushed face
- Headaches
- Irritability
- Loss of appetite
- Low back pain
- Low blood pressure

- Nosebleeds
- Poor concentration
- Recurring urinary tract infections

- Sinus pressure
- Soreness of muscles and joints
- Water retention

More serious cases of dehydration can also produce chronic pain, fever, and a rapid heart rate. If several of these symptoms sound familiar to you, insufficient water intake may be contributing to your inability to shed those extra pounds.

HOW DOES INSUFFICIENT WATER INTAKE CONTRIBUTE TO WEIGHT GAIN?

Insufficient water consumption has a number of consequences for your body that can lead to weight gain, both directly and indirectly. As you know, water is crucial for your body to function properly, and one of the many processes for which water is needed is the burning of fat. The liver is the organ that metabolizes fat, and the kidneys strain waste products and toxins from the bloodstream. When your water intake is inadequate, your kidneys cannot function at an optimal level, and additional support from the liver is required. The liver must therefore work twice as hard to both perform its own set of physiological functions *and* aid the kidneys. As a result, more of the fat you consume is stored rather than burned off, causing weight gain.

The failure to drink enough water can also affect your appetite. Because H_2O is a natural appetite suppressant, drinking a glass of water with or in between meals can fill you up more quickly and keep your hunger at bay. Insufficient water intake can cause your stomach to feel empty, and the natural response is to reach for chips, cookies, or some other snack that will satisfy your appetite—when all your body may really need is water. Regularly mistaking your body's thirst signals for hunger will also lead to weight gain, especially if your snacks are high in calories.

Another way insufficient water intake contributes to weight gain has to do with your muscles. When you're dehydrated, your blood volume decreases and less oxygen reaches your muscle tissues, causing you to feel tired and sluggish. Less water reaching your muscles also reduces their pliability, often leading to aches and joint soreness. This combination—achiness and flagging energy—may not only deter you from participating in physical activity, but also impair your body's performance during exercise. An unfortunate but common result is weight gain.

Insufficient water intake also causes water retention, bloating, constipation, digestive difficulties, and the buildup of toxins in your body, all of which can hinder weight-loss progress. If you want to get rid of excess weight, fitting in your 8 to 9 cups a day is key.

HOW DO YOU DETERMINE IF YOU DRINK ENOUGH WATER?

Even if you are not experiencing the symptoms listed on page 56, it's still possible that you're not drinking as much water as your body needs. Most people do not calculate how much they're drinking each day, and even fewer people pay attention to the color of their urine—which is the easiest way to gauge your water intake. Ideally, your urine should be colorless or a pale shade of yellow, as this indicates that the chemicals produced during the breakdown of your food have been watered down. Urine that is dark yellow in color, however, is a sign that your body requires more water than you are supplying.

Still, it is possible to drink *too much* water. The medical term for this potentially fatal condition is *hyponatremia*, which occurs when water begins to dilute the blood and flush out nutrients that your body requires. To avoid "overdosing" on water, never attempt to drink your entire daily requirement at once, but rather spread your glasses out throughout the day so that your body is consistently hydrated. In addition, people who have adrenal or kidney problems, or who have been prescribed diuretics by their doctor, should check with their physician before increasing their daily water intake.

WHAT CAN YOU DO TO LOSE WEIGHT?

Fitting in 8 to 9 glasses of water every day can seem like a burden and a chore—which may be why so many people neglect to do so. But by following some of the simple tips listed below, you'll find that meeting your daily water requirement is both effortless and energizing:

• Drink a glass of water as soon as you wake up to rehydrate.

• Plan your glasses of water, and stick to your schedule: Drink a glass before leaving for work, before or after lunch, during your mid-afternoon slump, with your dinner, and so on. Keep in mind that it's best to stop drinking water about two hours before bedtime to ensure restful sleep, unbroken by trips to the bathroom.

- Carry a water bottle with you when you're on the go, or keep it on your desk to drink throughout the workday and refill as needed. If possible, use a water bottle that is the size of your water intake requirement for the day—then you'll be sure when you've meet your goal.

- Use a filter to purify your water. This will enhance water's taste, making it more appealing to you, and will help remove chemicals and potentially harmful toxins.

- When you become bored with water's lack of flavor, add a squirt of lemon or lime or a small amount of fruit juice for some taste and a little variety.

- Increase your intake of water-rich foods like watermelon (92 percent water), tomatoes (95 percent), and yogurt (85 percent). Grapefruit, broccoli, apples, and eggs also have high water content.

- Remember to add a cup of water to your daily requirement every time you drink a cup of coffee or another diuretic beverage. Add about two cups of water to make up for moderate to intense exercise.

With these guidelines and some determination, drinking water will become a basic part of your daily routine. Once you're in the habit of drinking 8 to 9 glasses (or more) each day, you will feel rejuvenated and healthy. More important, you may find that those unwanted pounds gradually melt away.

CONCLUSION

The connection between weight loss and water intake is hard to deny. Drinking water is one of the healthiest and most natural ways to burn fat efficiently, satisfy your appetite, and tone your muscles, and each of these functions goes a long way when it comes to losing weight. With a few simple adjustments to your lifestyle, you can start fitting in the ounces your body needs, and maybe even begin to enjoy water's refreshing taste.

On the other hand, insufficient water intake may be just one of several factors that are keeping you from shedding pounds. If you take steps to increase your water consumption and still are unable to lose weight, be sure to explore the other chapters in this book, each of which examines a specific lifestyle issue, health problem, or biochemical factor that may be affecting your efforts to reduce. Once you have identified the contributing factors, turn to Chapter 20, "Putting It All Together," which will help you create an integrated weight-loss program that is suited to your needs.

PART II

Health Problems

Introduction
to Part II

Some health problems are easy to spot. A sore throat and fever, for instance, immediately tell you that something is very wrong so that you quickly seek medical treatment. In other cases, your doctor may discover a problem through a routine examination or test. A number of health disorders, however, are not as simple to detect but can still have a profound effect on your well-being. Food allergies, chronic inflammation, thyroid hormone insufficiency, toxic buildup, or an overgrowth of yeast can take their toll over time by causing fatigue, body aches and pains, and many other problems—including weight gain, obesity, and the inability to shed pounds.

Part II examines five common health disorders that have been linked to excess weight. In each chapter, you'll learn about the problem being examined, read a comprehensive list of symptoms, and discover how this issue can lead to unwanted pounds. You will then find guidelines for determining if this problem is compromising your health. Finally, you'll discover the many approaches you can take—including diet, exercise, and nutritional supplements—to treat this illness and help your body achieve a healthy weight.

If you are wondering if an undetected health problem is stopping you from losing weight, take the self-test presented on page 63. If your answers indicate that an underlying disorder may be at fault, Chapters 8 through 12 will guide you in taking the first important steps toward a healthier, slimmer body.

HEALTH PROBLEM QUESTIONNAIRE

This test was designed to help you determine if health issues, such as food allergies or chronic inflammation, may be hindering your attempts to lose weight. For each of the following questions, check the box that most accurately applies to you. When you have completed the questionnaire, count the number of times you answered "Often." If you checked this answer more than ten times, chances are that one or more disorders are compromising your ability to lose unwanted pounds. Read Chapters 8 through 12 to learn why your answers may indicate a problem, and how treating some common health disorders can make it easier to lose weight.

	Seldom	Sometimes	Often
1. Do you have cravings for a particular food?	☐	☐	☐
2. Do you have nasal congestion?	☐	☐	☐
3. Do you suffer from coughing?	☐	☐	☐
4. Do you have shortness of breath?	☐	☐	☐
5. Do you have heart palpitations (racing or pounding heart)?	☐	☐	☐
6. Do you experience stomach cramps, heartburn, or nausea?	☐	☐	☐
7. Do you feel depressed?	☐	☐	☐
8. Do you feel disoriented or confused?	☐	☐	☐
9. Do you experience anxiety and panic attacks?	☐	☐	☐
10. Do you have difficulty concentrating on tasks?	☐	☐	☐
11. Do you have body aches and pains?	☐	☐	☐
12. Do you experience fluid retention?	☐	☐	☐

	Seldom	Sometimes	Often
13. Do you have skin disorders such as dermatitis, eczema, or psoriasis?	☐	☐	☐
14. Do you have canker sores?	☐	☐	☐
15. Do you have bad breath (halitosis)?	☐	☐	☐
16. Do you smoke?	☐	☐	☐
17. Do you spend time near industrial plants, areas of high vehicle traffic, or toxic substances?	☐	☐	☐
18. Do you eat processed foods?	☐	☐	☐
19. Do you experience painful intercourse?	☐	☐	☐
20. Do you have a decreased interest in sex?	☐	☐	☐

TOTALS _____   _____ _____

8

Food Allergies

Have you ever suddenly found yourself sniffling and sneezing without any sign of a typical allergen like pollen? Have you ever become watery-eyed and congested without being anywhere near cat or dog hair? Perhaps hives appeared on your face without any obvious cause. To understand your problem, it may be time to look at the food on your plate. As you may know, food allergies can cause any of the conditions mentioned above, as well as a handful of even more severe symptoms. But are you aware that food allergies can also make you *crave* the very foods that create an allergic reaction? The truth is that food allergies could be the very reason you're overeating, putting on unwanted pounds, and finding it so hard to lose weight.

Sixty percent of Americans suffer from some sort of adverse reaction to food. Some food allergies cause severe reactions in certain people, including difficulty breathing, low blood pressure, and even death. Other food allergies produce milder symptoms, such as itchy skin or eyes. Unfortunately, the chemical reactions that attempt to eliminate a food allergen from your body may also make you eat more of that particular allergenic food, ultimately resulting in weight gain. And if allergies aren't the culprit, food intolerances—another type of food sensitivity that has similar consequences—may be. These issues can cause not only physical symptoms but also psychological ones, including depression and anxiety, which may further contribute to your inability to lose weight.

Food allergies are a complex subject that health practitioners are only now beginning to understand. Thankfully, there are commonsense ways to avoid this problem and alleviate the sensitivities you didn't even know you had. After you learn a little bit about allergies and intolerances, the next thing you must do, of course, is recognize their symptoms. In doing so you will be able to narrow down which foods might be affecting you.

WHAT ARE FOOD ALLERGIES?

Allergies occur when your body shows a hypersensitivity to a normally harmless substance in the environment. When you come into contact with this substance, also called an *allergen*, it triggers your body's immune system to release compounds called *histamines*. These histamines widen your blood vessels, causing inflammation, which allows proteins known as *antibodies* to enter tissue and neutralize the allergen that they mistakenly consider a dangerous invader. This overreaction of your immune system can manifest itself outwardly with physical signs, including a runny nose, wheezing, or a rash, to name but a few.

While allergic reactions are most often caused when a person comes into contact with airborne substances such as dust or pollen, your body can also be set off by certain proteins in food. The most common allergenic foods are milk, eggs, peanuts, tree nuts (including almonds, cashews, and walnuts), seafood, shellfish, soy, and wheat, although the possibilities are numerous. Reactions to eating allergenic foods can range from mild sneezing and coughing, as are seen with airborne allergens, to a life-threatening condition called *anaphylaxis*. Anaphylaxis symptoms can include a swelling of the throat, shortness of breath, and even the loss of consciousness, all of which may end in death if not treated quickly.

Sometimes a negative reaction to food, however, may be due to an intolerance of that food rather than an allergy. Unlike a food allergy, which causes your immune system to see a particular food as a foreign poison to be eliminated, a food intolerance merely means that your body lacks the necessary enzymes to break down that food properly. Although it can produce many of the same symptoms as food allergies, reactions to food intolerance are usually less severe but more delayed. They are uncomfortable but not life-threatening. Both food intolerances and food allergies, however, can affect your weight. To combat the problem, your best bet is to determine the foods that irritate you and remove them from your diet. In order to accomplish that task, you must first recognize the symptoms of these conditions.

WHAT ARE THE SYMPTOMS OF FOOD ALLERGIES?

The amount of an allergenic food necessary to cause a reaction differs, depending on the person. The severity of symptoms also ranges from mild to life-threatening. Generally, however, a food allergy will result in one or more of the following physical signs:

- Abdominal pain
- Anal itching
- Anaphylaxis
- Anemia
- Backache
- Breathing difficulties
- Canker sores
- Chest pain
- Cracks at corner of mouth
- Dark circles under eyes
- Diarrhea
- Dizziness
- Eczema
- Fatigue
- Fluid retention
- Food cravings
- Frequent urination
- Gas
- Headaches
- Heart palpitation
- Heartburn
- Hives
- Hoarseness
- Itchy, watery eyes
- Itchy skin
- Low blood pressure
- Muscle aches
- Nasal congestion
- Nausea
- Persistent cough
- Rash or hives
- Reddened earlobes, eyes, or cheeks
- Ringing in ears (tinnitus)
- Sniffling and sneezing
- Stomach cramps
- Tension headaches
- Tremors
- Wrinkles under eyes

Amazingly, your thoughts and actions may also be governed by allergic reactions. Research has begun to link allergies to a number of mental and emotional symptoms, including:

- Anxiety
- Attention deficit hyperactivity disorder (ADHD)
- Brain fog (confusion)
- Compulsive behavior
- Depression
- Disorientation
- Dyslexia
- Emotional outbursts
- Epilepsy
- Irritability
- Lethargy
- Memory loss
- Mood swings
- Panic attacks
- Paranoia
- Restlessness
- Weepiness

While food intolerances share many of the same symptoms as food allergies, the majority of complaints center on the digestive tract, as the problem is one of digestion. You may be suffering from an intolerance of a certain food if you experience one or more of the following symptoms after eating:

- Diarrhea
- Gas, cramps, or bloating
- Headaches
- Heartburn

- Irritability or nervousness
- Nausea
- Stomach pain
- Vomiting

If you have been experiencing any of these symptoms but cannot find a reason why, you may be suffering from a food allergy or intolerance, both of which can contribute to unintended weight gain.

HOW DO FOOD ALLERGIES CONTRIBUTE TO WEIGHT GAIN?

As if headaches and heart palpitations weren't enough, food allergies can actually play a role in weight gain. If you frequently find yourself craving certain foods for no reason, it could be that you are mildly allergic to those foods and don't realize it. Unfortunately, the same chemical reactions set into motion by your body's immune system after eating an allergenic food can give you a slight "high" feeling. Understandably, this feeling causes cravings for the allergenic food. And, like a drug addict, you undergo symptoms of withdrawal when that food is taken away. To avoid withdrawal, you tend to overindulge in the food, putting on pounds in the process.

In addition to the problem of cravings, research has shown that allergies disrupt an area of the brain called the *limbic* region, which regulates hunger, and also interfere with proper neurotransmitter function, which can lead to increased body mass. (To learn more about neurotransmitters and weight gain, see Chapter 18.) Finally, the inflammatory reaction of your immune system causes your body to retain water and contributes to your inability to lose weight. (To learn about inflammation and weight gain, see Chapter 9.)

So if you catch yourself with the urge to eat certain foods, or find yourself overeating for reasons you cannot explain, it may be time to determine if you are suffering from a food allergy.

HOW DO YOU DETERMINE IF YOU HAVE FOOD ALLERGIES?

Because you typically eat a combination of foods during a meal, it can be difficult to pinpoint the exact food to which you are allergic or intolerant. Your doctor can test your blood for antibodies called *immunoglobulin E*, or IgE, to determine possible allergies, or antibodies called *immunoglobulin G*, or IgG, to determine possible intolerances. Neither of these tests, however, is completely reliable. As a result, your doctor will most likely ask you to eliminate the most commonly recognized allergens from your diet and reintroduce each one individually, paying attention to your body's response. Cutting out the foods you seem to desire most, as well as foods such as milk, eggs, peanuts, tree nuts, seafood, shellfish, soy, and wheat, would be a good start in your search for the culprit.

The elimination method may sound like a real chore, but you will thank yourself for having gone through it once you are free of food allergies and intolerances. Sometimes, you can reintroduce a problem food into your diet in small amounts after three to four months, so you may not need to deny yourself a certain food completely.

WHAT CAN YOU DO TO LOSE WEIGHT?

After all the hard work of getting tested and following an elimination diet to determine your food allergies and intolerances, the solution to your problem is fairly straightforward. Basically, you need to avoid the foods that are causing the negative reactions in your body. As previously mentioned, not all allergies require total elimination of a food. You may still be able to eat what you like if you are willing to reduce your portion. Once you've removed or significantly reduced a problem food from your diet, you should begin to notice a difference in your ability to lose weight. The pounds of retained fluid will be the first to go, while your lack of extreme cravings will curb your tendency to overeat, contributing to further weight loss. You should feel better physically and mentally, as your system is no longer producing all those troublesome chemicals in response to your diet.

CONCLUSION

Experiencing symptoms such as coughing, dizziness, and irritability without an explanation can be utterly frustrating. Having inexplicable cravings for foods that cause these symptoms without your knowledge may seem like a cruel joke—especially when you're trying to lose weight. But now that you understand food allergies and your body's response to them, you need not feel depressed and helpless. There are methods to determine which foods affect you, and an effective way to prevent those foods from doing any more damage to your lifestyle and waistline. Dietary modification can eliminate food allergies and intolerances, helping you rid yourself of extra pounds.

Food allergies, however, may not be your only hurdle on the road to weight loss. If you address this problem but still can't lose weight, be sure to explore the other chapters in this book, each of which examines a specific lifestyle issue, health disorder, or biochemical factor that may be affecting your efforts to reduce. Once you have identified the contributing factors, turn to Chapter 20, "Putting It All Together," which will help you create an integrated weight-loss program that is suited to your needs.

9

Chronic Inflammation

Like everyone else, you've probably experienced inflammation many times in your life. When you accidentally stubbed your toe on a piece of furniture, for example, your toe probably became red, swollen, and painful. Finally, the swelling decreased and your toe healed. The physical symptoms of swelling and pain—part of the process known as acute inflammation—were of short duration and were actually a necessary stage of your recovery. But inflammation is not always a limited, health-promoting event. Sometimes, this physical response becomes chronic, continuing despite the fact that it is not needed to promote healing or because healing has failed to occur. This can lead to numerous disorders, including obesity and the inability to lose weight.

Experts believe that chronic inflammation is now a major problem in our society, primarily due to our diet. The foods that we typically eat promote both inflammation and weight gain, and the excess body fat that results from weight gain leads to yet more inflammation, creating a downward spiral. Fortunately, the inflammatory process can be avoided and even reversed. By making a wise choice of foods and supplementing your diet with carefully selected nutrients—and, perhaps, a little more physical activity—you can eliminate chronic inflammation and enjoy a healthier, slimmer body.

WHAT IS CHRONIC INFLAMMATION?

To understand chronic inflammation, it's helpful to first take a closer look at *acute inflammation*, the body's normal response to tissue damage. This process is designed to defend the body against harmful substances like bacteria, eliminate dead or dying tissue, and promote the renewal of healthy tissue.

When body tissue becomes injured—say, by a cut from a kitchen knife or the invasion of bacteria—there is a release of chemicals such as histamines and prostaglandins, which widen the blood vessels in the area, increasing blood flow. A side effect of this process is the visible swelling and redness that occur after an injury, as well as a feeling of heat and increased pain from the pressure exerted on nerves by the swollen tissues. The released chemicals signal the migration of white blood cells, the body's defense cells, to the injured area. These cells neutralize harmful bacteria and actually ingest the dead cells so that new ones may grow. Following this, the repair process begins and swelling and other signs of inflammation subside. Eventually, all damaged tissue is replaced by healthy tissue.

Without acute inflammation, wounds and infections would never heal. But this response is a tightly orchestrated event that is designed to continue only long enough to protect the tissue from further harm and initiate the healing process. Sometimes inflammation persists beyond this point, or the process is triggered even when there is no injury or invasion of harmful agents, such as bacteria. In this situation, called *chronic inflammation*, the body continues to destroy its own tissue—not only unhealthy tissue, but also healthy tissue. If you think of chronic inflammatory diseases such as rheumatoid arthritis and gout, you can visualize just how destructive (and painful) this situation can be. In recent years, researchers have also linked inflammation to less obvious disorders. By looking at the body's level of c-reactive protein (CRP), a major marker of inflammation, they have found that the inflammatory response plays an important part in heart attacks, type 2 diabetes, Alzheimer's disease, and even cancer. They have also begun to understand the relationship between weight gain and inflammation.

Why is chronic inflammation now such a pervasive problem? For the most part, researchers blame the standard American diet, sometimes referred to as SAD. A diet high in sugar, high in trans fats, high in omega-6 fatty acids, and low in omega-3 fatty acids creates chronic inflammation in the body. (To learn more about good and bad fats, see the inset on page 73.) Foods high on the glycemic index (GI)—foods that break down quickly during digestion, causing a surge in blood sugar—also appear to play a role in inflammation. In one study of women with diabetes, CRP inflammatory levels were 32 percent higher when subjects ate high-GI foods. (For information on blood sugar, see Chapter 16. For information on high- and low-GI foods, see page 156.) Finally, food sensitivities and intolerances—unpleasant reactions to food, usually as the result of the digestive

A Primer on Good and Bad Fats

On page 72 of this chapter, you learned that certain bad fats can lead to chronic inflammation. But certain fats are actually necessary for good health and serve to *reduce* inflammation. Let's take a look at some important good and bad fats.

Trans fats, also known as *trans-fatty acids*, are man-made substances created when liquid vegetable oils are hydrogenated to make them more solid (like butter), more shelf-stable, and more useful in the production of baked goods. Studies have shown that these fats increase LDL, the "bad cholesterol"; lower HDL, the "good cholesterol"; increase triglycerides; and promote chronic inflammation. To avoid these harmful substances, choose whole, natural foods—trans fats are mostly found in margarine, crackers, cookies, chips, doughnuts, and pastries—and look for the "No Trans Fats" label on prepared items.

There are two types of *essential fatty acids (EFAs)—omega-3* and *omega-6*. Although both are needed for good health, the American diet tends to be much heavier in omega-6 fatty acids than omega-3. Since omega-6 fats promote inflammation and omega-3 fats decrease it, you can relieve many inflammation-related conditions by limiting your intake of omega-6-rich foods and adding more foods rich in omega-3. The following table, which lists foods high in each of the two EFAs, should help you get your fatty acid intake into balance. You can also reduce inflammation by taking omega-3 EFAs in supplement form (see the table on page 80).

FOODS RICH IN ESSENTIAL FATTY ACIDS

Omega-3 Fatty Acids	Omega-6 Fatty Acids
Beans	Corn oil
Broccoli and other dark green vegetables	Cottonseed oil
	Flaxseed oil
Canola oil	Safflower oil
Cold-water fatty fish, including albacore tuna, herring, lake trout, mackerel, salmon, sardines	Salad dressings and mayonnaise made from the oils listed above.
Flaxseed oil	Soybean oil
Soybean oil	Sunflower oil

tract's inability to metabolize a substance such as lactose (lactose intolerance) or gluten (gluten intolerance)—can create chronic, low-level inflammation and fluid retention.

WHAT ARE THE SYMPTOMS OF CHRONIC INFLAMMATION?

Symptoms of chronic inflammation vary, depending partly on the area of the body where the runaway reaction is taking hold. Directly below, you will find general symptoms of chronic inflammation. Following this are groups of health disorders that involve inflammation, and therefore indicate its presence. Be aware, though, that this type of inflammation usually takes place without the obvious symptoms characteristic of acute inflammation. There may be no swollen, painful joints. There may be no redness. In many cases, only the presence of inflammatory disorders will clue you into this problem.

General Signs of Chronic Inflammation

- Body aches and pains
- Chronic diarrhea
- Chronic indigestion
- Dry eyes
- Fluid retention
- Frequent infection
- Nasal congestion
- Shortness of breath
- Skin outbreaks
- Stiffness of joints
- Swelling of joints
- Weight gain/obesity

Allergic Reactions

- Celiac disease/gluten intolerance
- Food allergies
- Rhinitis (inflammation of the nasal mucous membranes)

Arthritic Conditions

- Gout
- Osteoarthritis
- Rheumatoid arthritis

Autoimmune Diseases

- Lupus erythematosus
- Multiple sclerosis

Cancer

- Breast
- Colon
- Lung
- Prostate
- Stomach

Cardiovascular Disorders

- Coronary artery disease
- Hypertension (high blood pressure)
- Myocarditis (inflammation of the heart muscle)

Dental Problems

- Gingivitis (inflammation of the gums)
- Periodontitis (infection of the gums)

Eye Disorders

- Conjunctivitis (pink eye)
- Uveitis (inflammation of the middle layer of the eye)

Gastrointestinal Problems

- Crohn's disease
- Diverticulitis
- Gastritis (inflammation of the stomach lining)
- Irritable bowel syndrome (IBS)
- Ulcerative colitis
- Ulcers

Glandular Disorders

- Diabetes
- Thyroiditis (inflammation of the thyroid gland)

Injuries

- Bruises
- Bursitis
- Muscle strains
- Tendonitis

Neurological Disorders

- Alzheimer's disease

Respiratory Pulmonary Disorders

- Asthma
- Bronchitis
- Chronic obstructive pulmonary disease (COPD)

Skin Disorders

- Acne
- Dermatitis
- Eczema
- Psoriasis

If several of the symptoms in the above lists sound familiar to you, perhaps chronic inflammation is contributing to your weight-loss problem.

HOW DOES CHRONIC INFLAMMATION CONTRIBUTE TO WEIGHT GAIN?

It is a vicious cycle: Gaining too much weight promotes inflammation, and inflammation promotes obesity.

It's important to understand that adipose tissue—body fat, in other words—is not inactive, but secretes a host of chemicals, including CRP, the marker for inflammation discussed earlier in the chapter. This is one of the chief ways in which increased weight fuels the inflammatory process. In turn, inflammation has a profound effect on metabolism by making the brain and body resistant to the normal weight-regulating hormones, including leptin, insulin, and cortisol. By affecting leptin—the hormone that lets you know you are full—inflammation causes you to overeat. By tampering with insulin and cortisol, the inflammatory process prevents the breakdown of fat and causes fat cells to actually grow, hindering your attempts to lose excess pounds.

Inflammation can also support weight gain in more subtle ways. If you look at the lists on pages 74 to 76, you'll see that the many disorders related to chronic inflammation include arthritis, asthma, and bronchitis. All of these health problems tend to limit physical activity to some degree, and as physical activity decreases, pounds tend to accumulate.

HOW DO YOU DETERMINE IF YOU HAVE CHRONIC INFLAMMATION?

As already mentioned, chronic inflammation usually doesn't announce itself with easy-to-spot symptoms such as swelling and redness. But if you have reason to believe that this disorder is compromising your health, your doctor may order one of the following tests. Your primary care physician can arrange any of the first three tests. The last one—the inflammatory cytokine profile—would be ordered by a physician who specializes in immunology or in metabolic and anti-aging medicine.

- **C-Reactive Protein (CRP) Test.** This simple blood test measures the body's level of CRP—a protein that is present in inflammation. This test is sometimes used after surgery, after treatment for infection, or to check the risk of developing coronary artery disease by measuring inflammation in the arteries. Although this analysis is fairly accurate, a low CRP level does not necessarily mean that there is no inflammation.

- **Erythrocyte Sedimentation Rate (ESR).** This blood test measures the rate at which red blood cells (erythrocytes) fall to the bottom of a test tube that is left standing upright. When certain inflammation-marking proteins cover the erythrocytes, the cells stick together and fall more quickly, indicating inflammation.

- **Fasting Blood Insulin Test.** This test, designed to screen for diabetes and heart disease, is also a marker for inflammation. The higher your insulin levels, the greater your body's inflammatory response.

- **Inflammatory Cytokine Profile.** Considered by many to be the ultimate test for measuring inflammation, it screens the blood for certain protein molecules (cytokines)—chiefly, interleukins, interferon, and tumor necrosis factor—that the body produces as part of the inflammatory process.

If any of the above tests show that an inflammatory condition is present, the doctor may order further tests to identify the cause of the problem so that appropriate treatment can be prescribed.

WHAT CAN YOU DO TO LOSE WEIGHT?

If you have reason to believe that chronic inflammation is preventing you from successfully losing weight—and may be contributing to other health disorders, as well—you can do a great deal to control the inflammatory process so that weight gain becomes easier. As you might have guessed, a good first step is to modify your diet so that it limits sugars, trans fats, and omega-6 fatty acids, and provides a healthy amount of the anti-inflammatory omega-3 fatty acids. Just as important, you want to emphasize foods that are lower on the glycemic index. (For a discussion of the glycemic index, see page 156 in Chapter 16.)

Although experts have offered different diets to reduce inflammation, most agree that the ideal plan would be close to the Mediterranean diet, which appears to have powerful anti-inflammatory properties. In fact, studies have shown that even *one day* on the Mediterranean diet lowers levels of the inflammatory marker CRP. The Mediterranean diet is also known to promote the loss of weight. Following are the basic guidelines for a healthy Mediterranean-style eating plan:

- As much as possible, stick to fresh, healthy foods such as fruits and vegetables, whole grains, nuts and seeds, legumes (beans), seafood, yogurt, and olive oil.

- Limit your portion sizes. This diet focuses on small portions of high-quality foods that are satisfying due to the high fiber content of the produce coupled with the delicious flavors of ingredients such as olive oil and nuts.

- Include fats, but keep them healthy by getting them from olive oil, nuts, avocados, and fatty fish such as salmon, tuna, trout, and sardines. By limiting processed and packaged foods, you'll automatically reduce your consumption of inflammatory trans fats.

- In general, keep your consumption of red meat and poultry as low as you possibly can. The healthiest Mediterranean diets are nearly vegetarian, with lots of vegetables, beans, whole grains, and fish, and very little meat. Feel free to enjoy servings of lamb, though, as this particular meat—an important part of some Mediterranean diets—is high in inflammation-fighting omega-3 fatty acids.

- Eat your grains whole. Bread, couscous, pasta, and polenta are all beneficial foods as long as long as portions are modest and the grains have not been refined.

- If health permits, enjoy a little wine with dinner—but only a little! Mediterranean wine glasses are small, and people typically drink only three to six ounces of wine with their evening meal.

- For dessert, enjoy fruit—not sugar-laden cookies, cakes, or ice cream.

If you suspect that food sensitivities or intolerances may be contributing to chronic inflammation, but you haven't been able to pinpoint the food or foods that are causing the problem, your doctor may recommend that you eliminate the foods most commonly responsible for intolerances from your diet and then reintroduce each one individually, paying attention to your body's response. Once you are able to identify and avoid the trigger foods, you may be able to reduce inflammation and begin to shed pounds. (For more about identifying food intolerances, see the inset "Do You Have a Food Intolerance?" below.)

In addition to modifying your diet to include only anti-inflammatory foods, consider taking supplements such as omega-3 essential fatty acids,

Do You Have a Food Intolerance?

If you read Chapter 8, you know that a food intolerance is different from a food allergy in that the immune system is not involved. Instead, the body is unable to break down the food properly, usually because it lacks the enzymes necessary to do so. There are many different types of food intolerances. Most common are sensitivities to the following substances:

- Food preservatives and additives (found in processed foods)
- Gluten (found in wheat, oats, barley, and rye)
- Lactose (found in milk and milk products)
- Tyramine (found in aged cheese, avocados, beer, chocolate, pickled herring, raspberries, sausage, wine, and yeast)

Food intolerances and sensitivities can cause a wide range of symptoms, which may affect you on a constant basis or only from time to time. They can include but are not limited to:

- Digestive problems such as nausea, vomiting, diarrhea, constipation, flatulence (gas), and irritable bowel syndrome (IBS)
- Skin problems such as hives, rashes, psoriasis, and eczema
- Weight gain
- Yeast infections

If symptoms indicate that you may have an intolerance or sensitivity to certain foods, an effective means of pinpointing the problem is an elimination diet, which is explained on page 69. This can help you establish a healthier way of eating, free of foods that can lead to inflammation and related health disorders.

which can help reduce the inflammatory response and alleviate some of the unpleasant symptoms associated with inflammation. The table found below suggests dosages and presents considerations you should keep in mind when taking these substances. Be sure to consult a physician before using these supplements.

SUPPLEMENTS TO TREAT INFLAMMATION

Supplement	Dosage	Considerations
Bromelain	250 mg twice a day.	Bromelain is a protease, an enzyme that dissolves protein. Do not take this supplement if you are allergic to pineapple.
Catechin green tea	1 cup three times a day.	If tea causes heartburn or acid reflux, drink it with a meal.
Garlic (*Allium sativum*)	400 mg twice a day.	Do not take if you are on a blood-thinning medication.
Ginger root (*Zingiber officinale*)	500 mg twice a day.	Do not take if you are on a blood-thinning medication or NSAIDs. If you have allergies, cardiac problems, central nervous system problems, or renal problems, consult with your health-care provider before taking ginger.
Ginkgo (*Ginkgo biloba*)	120 mg once a day.	Do not take if you are on a blood-thinning medication.
Glucosamine	500 to 1,000 mg three times a day.*	Do not take if you are allergic to shellfish. Consult with your health-care provider if you have diabetes, because glucosamine can alter blood sugar levels.
Grape seed extract and pycnogenol	50 mg twice a day.	Consult with your health-care provider if you have diabetes or hypoglycemia (low blood sugar); take cholesterol-lowering medications; have a history of bleeding or clotting disorders; or take anticoagulant medications, NSAIDs, anti-platelet medications, blood pressure medications, or medications that stimulate or suppress the immune system.
Methylsulfonyl-methane (MSM)	1,000 to 3,000 mg three times a day.*	Use with caution if you have kidney disease, liver disease, or an ulcer. High doses can deplete your body of other vitamins in the B complex.

Omega-3 essential fatty acids EPA/DHA (fish oil)	2,000 to 10,000 mg once a day.*	In dosages above 4,000 mg, may cause the blood to thin. Do not take more than 4,000 mg a day if you are using a blood-thinning medication.
Quercetin	200 to 500 mg once a day.*	If supplement causes heartburn or acid reflux, take the dose with a meal.
Trans-resveratrol	200 mg once a day.	To avoid additives such as caffeine, look for a product that is 99 percent trans-resveratrol.
Turmeric curcuminoids	300 mg twice a day.	May cause an upset stomach or heartburn. In susceptible people, may increase the risk of kidney stones.

*To choose an appropriate dose, see page 199 for information on dosage ranges.

Finally, be aware that exercise is a safe and inexpensive form of anti-inflammatory medicine. When properly performed, exercise actually releases substances that control inflammation and result in the repair and regeneration of strong, healthy tissues. Some experts believe that the absence of physical movement in the modern world has played a part in the increase of inflammation-related disorders such as asthma, heart disease, diabetes, and cancer. By making exercise part of your life, you can help normalize your body's inflammatory response and transform chronic inflammation into healing. (To learn more about the role of exercise in the weight-loss process, turn to Chapter 2.) Just keep in mind that vigorous exercise can result in an inflammatory response. Moderation is the key, so limit your exercise to three times a week.

CONCLUSION

Chronic inflammation is now recognized as an underlying factor in a host of disorders, from coronary heart disease to cancer to obesity. If you feel that this all-too-common problem is preventing you from shedding pounds, there are numerous steps you can take to reverse the condition. In many cases, dietary modifications and appropriate nutritional supplementation—helped, ideally, by exercise—can calm inflammation, improve your overall health, and enable you to reach your desired weight.

On the other hand, chronic inflammation may be just one of several factors that are keeping you from slimming down. If you take steps to treat this disorder and are still unable to lose weight, be sure to explore the other chapters in this book, each of which examines a specific lifestyle issue, health problem, or biochemical factor that may be affecting your efforts to reduce. Once you have identified the contributing factors, turn to Chapter 20, "Putting It All Together," which will help you create an integrated weight-loss program that is suited to your needs.

10

Thyroid Hormone Dysfunction

You're cutting back on sweets. You're exercising. You're doing everything possible to lose weight, but for some reason, those extra pounds just aren't coming off. You're feeling tired, sluggish, and depressed, but simply chalk it up to your weight problem. A friend says that maybe you've got a thyroid disorder, but you don't believe her. It sounds too much like an excuse—like saying you're "big-boned." But what if your friend is right?

The truth is that thyroid dysfunction *may* actually be the hidden cause of your problem. Thyroid hormones can have a major effect on your waistline. Improper thyroid hormone levels can add pounds to your body while also making it difficult for you to lose weight. In addition, this disorder can lead to a large number of other physical and psychological conditions, which are often dismissed as symptoms of merely being overweight. Thyroid dysfunction is an extremely common illness that affects over 20 million Americans—a statistic that is even higher than the rate of diabetes in the United States. Identifying and correcting a thyroid problem could be your first step towards a happier and healthier life. By shining a light on the subject, you may finally understand what has been preventing you from reaching your ideal weight.

WHAT IS THYROID HORMONE DYSFUNCTION?

In order to understand thyroid hormone dysfunction, you need to know what the thyroid is, as well as what it does in your body. The thyroid is one of the largest and most important glands of your body's hormonal system. Located in the lower part of your neck, this gland secretes two hormones: *triiodothyronine*, or T_3, and *thyroxine*, or T_4. These hormones play a role in countless vital functions, one of which is *metabolism*—the conversion of oxygen and calories to energy.

The creation of thyroid hormones is a three-step process. First, your hypothalamus generates *thyrotropin-releasing hormone,* or TRH, which stimulates your pituitary gland to produce thyroid-stimulating hormone, also known as TSH. TSH then causes your thyroid to synthesize T_3 and T_4 from the essential trace element iodine and the amino acid tyrosine. In order to maintain the correct levels of T_3 and T_4, your pituitary gland increases the amount of TSH in your blood when thyroid hormones are low, and decreases it when thyroid hormones are high. Although T_3 is approximately five times as powerful as T_4, the thyroid manufactures about twenty times more T_4 than it does T_3. After these hormones are produced, they are released into the bloodstream and transported throughout your system, where they regulate the metabolism of every cell in your body.

When the production of thyroid hormones is normal, your body is helped to maintain a healthy weight. But when the thyroid is overactive, a condition called *hyperthyroidism,* it releases too much hormones, which speed your metabolism to an unhealthy level, causing unwanted weight loss. And when the thyroid is underactive, a condition known as *hypothyroidism,* it produces an insufficient amount of hormones, which slows your metabolism, making it much more difficult for your body to burn calories. Hypothyroidism, however, can result not only in weight gain but also in a number of other symptoms and disorders. Knowing what these symptoms are can help you figure out if you are, in fact, experiencing a thyroid problem.

WHAT ARE THE SYMPTOMS OF THYROID HORMONE DYSFUNCTION?

As discussed above, an underactive thyroid results in weight gain, as well as a host of other problems. Although you may not experience every one of these conditions, hypothyroidism often reveals itself through the following symptoms:

- Acne
- Allergies
- Anemia
- Anxiety
- Bladder and kidney infections
- Bone loss
- Brittle nails
- Carpal tunnel syndrome
- Cold hands and feet
- Cold intolerance

- Constipation
- Decreased reflexes
- Depression
- Difficulty concentrating
- Dizziness
- Down-turned mouth
- Droopy eyelids
- Dry, coarse, or thinning hair
- Dry, itchy ear canals
- Dull facial expression
- Easy bruising
- Eating disorders
- Erectile dysfunction
- Excess ear wax
- Fatigue
- Fluid retention
- Gallstones
- Goiter (enlarged thyroid gland)
- Headaches
- High cholesterol
- Hoarse, husky voice
- Increased appetite
- Insomnia
- Irritability
- Longer, heavier, or more frequent menstrual periods
- Loss of hair on legs, arms, or underarms
- Low blood pressure
- Low blood sugar
- Low sex drive
- Memory loss
- Muscle and joint pain
- Muscle weakness
- Nighttime incontinence
- Numbness and tingling of the extremities
- Poor circulation
- Poor night vision
- Puffy face
- Reduced heart rate
- Rough, dry skin
- Sleep apnea
- Slow speech
- Swollen legs, feet, hands, or abdomen
- Tennis elbow
- Thinning or loss of eyelashes
- Tinnitus
- Vitamin B_{12} deficiency
- Weight gain
- Yellow skin

If you are experiencing several of these problems, thyroid dysfunction may be a contributing factor to your inability to lose weight.

HOW DOES THYROID HORMONE DYSFUNCTION CONTRIBUTE TO WEIGHT GAIN?

As you are now aware, when your thyroid gland produces fewer T_3 and T_4 hormones, your metabolism slows down. This means that even if you watch what you eat, your body is less able to convert calories into energy. Those unused calories end up adding inches to your waistline. Slowly, over time, you can gain ten to fifteen pounds without even realizing it. Unfortunately, once you decide to lose those excess pounds, your lowered metabolism makes it much more difficult to shed weight than it used to be.

The combination of reduced metabolism and other symptoms of hypothyroidism makes losing weight seem like a losing battle. The depression and insomnia so often caused by hypothyroidism increase your likelihood of indulging in foods that are high in carbohydrates and fat, while the fatigue associated with an underactive thyroid makes it harder for you to engage in the physical activity necessary to burn off extra calories. (For more information on the effects of sleep deprivation and depression on weight gain, see Chapters 5 and 13, respectively.) The problem can be further compounded by a headache, difficulty concentrating, and muscle pain. Because many of these symptoms can be attributed to other causes, you should first get your thyroid checked to determine if it is, in fact, to blame.

HOW DO YOU DETERMINE IF YOU HAVE THYROID HORMONE DYSFUNCTION?

If you suspect that an underactive thyroid may be behind your weight gain and other health issues, it is time to see your doctor, who can perform a thyroid examination and order blood tests. These tests should measure your levels of T_3, T_4, TSH. Your doctor may also test for an elevated amount of thyroid antibodies in your system, which can stop thyroid hormones from successfully attaching to receptors, causing symptoms of decreased thyroid function even when your blood levels of T_3 and T_4 are adequate. Thyroid antibodies can be raised due to trauma, poor function of your gut, inflammation, or other problems.

Lastly, you should have your level of *reverse* T_3, or rT_3, checked. RT_3 is the inactive form of T_3. During the conversion of T_4 to T_3, sometimes rT_3 is produced instead. It is a normal occurrence, but too much rT_3 results in the same symptoms as an underactive thyroid, which is why it should be evaluated.

If your test results reveal that your thyroid is functioning poorly, the problem could be associated with certain nutritional deficiencies. For this reason, you should follow up by having your blood tested for sufficient levels of the following substances:

- Copper
- Iodine
- Iron
- Selenium

- Vitamin A
- Vitamin B_2
- Vitamin B_3
- Vitamin B_6

- Vitamin B_{12}
- Vitamin C
- Zinc

If your doctor determines that your thyroid hormones are low, he will most certainly prescribe hormone replacement medication to correct the problem. Dietary modifications and supplements may also be recommended to help boost your T_3 and T_4 levels naturally. By taking advantage of every possible treatment, you should have the right amount of thyroid hormones circulating in your blood before you know it. Then you can start dropping those extra pounds.

Factors That Contribute to Low Thyroid Hormone Levels

In addition to the nutritional deficiencies discussed above, there are a number of other factors that contribute to low levels of T_3 and T_4. Lifestyle choices, illness, and environmental toxins, for example, should all be considered when treating a poorly functioning thyroid. In particular, the following possibilities should be taken into account.

- Aging
- Alcohol abuse
- Dioxins
- Elevated lipoic acid
- Excess copper
- Heavy metal toxicity
- High fluoride levels

- Insufficient DHEA
- Medications, including beta blockers, birth control pills, chemotherapy, estrogen, lithium, phenytoin, and theophylline

- PCBs
- Pesticides
- Phthalates
- Radiation
- Stress
- Surgical removal of thyroid

WHAT CAN YOU DO TO LOSE WEIGHT?

Once hypothyroidism has been diagnosed, it is important that your doctor replace both hormones—T_3 and T_4—to get you back up and running correctly, as this strategy has been found to be much more effective than replacing T_4 alone.

Levothyroxine sodium (Synthroid) is a drug comprised only of T_4, while liothyronine sodium (Cytomel) is only T_3. It is possible to raise both hormone levels by combining levothyroxine sodium and liothyronine sodium according to the ratio suggested by your doctor. Your physician may also prescribe desiccated thyroid extract, which is made from dried and powdered animal thyroid glands, and contains T_3 and T_4 in a ratio of 4 to 1. Lastly, you could get both T_3 and T_4 in one pill by having your doctor prescribe compounded thyroid. In this way, your medication would be customized to meet your specific needs.

In addition to taking traditional thyroid drugs, consider using supplements to improve the conversion of T_4 to T_3 in your system. The table found below lists substances that help T_3 synthesis.

SUPPLEMENTS TO IMPROVE T_4 TO T_3 CONVERSION		
Supplement	Dosage	Consideration
Ashwagandha root	500 to 1,000 mg once a day.*	Do not take if you are pregnant. Possible side effects may include nausea, vomiting, and diarrhea.
B-complex vitamins	Choose a B-complex vitamin that provides 10 to 50 mg each of vitamins B_1, B_2, B_3, B_5, and B_6; 200 to 400 mcg of folic acid; and 250 to 500 mcg of B_{12}. Take twice a day.	Speak to your health-care provider before taking if you have diabetes, liver problems, or anemia. B-complex vitamins may interact with certain antibiotics and anti-seizure medications. Whenever taking a B-complex vitamin, always take a multivitamin as well.
Iodine	• 150 mcg a day for adults who are not pregnant. • 220 mcg a day for pregnant women To determine a personalized dosage, have your doctor measure your iodine levels.	Do not take iodine if you are allergic to shellfish.

Iron	• 10 mg once a day for men. • 15 mg once a day for premenopausal women. • 30 mg once a day for pregnant women.	Men over the age of fifty and meno-pausal women should not consume iron supplements unless instructed by their doctor. Ferrous sulfate can cause constipation and nausea. Blood thinners and certain other drugs are less absorbed when taken with iron, so speak to your doctor if you are on medication.
Melatonin	1 to 6 mg once a day, before bedtime.*	For ideal use, take thirty minutes before bedtime while in a dark room. Start by taking 1 mg and increase your dose as needed. People who are pregnant, take prescription steroids, or have depression, mental illness, leukemia, lymphoma, or an autoimmune disease should not take melatonin. Possible side effects include headache, fatigue, and nightmares.
Multivitamin, pharmaceutical-grade†	Follow the directions on the bottle.	Make sure to take only a pharmaceutical-grade multivitamin.
Potassium	To determine proper dosage, have your doctor measure your potassium levels.	Always take this supplement with water to prevent it from getting stuck in your throat and causing damage to your esophagus. Do not take potassium if you have kidney failure.
Selenium	100 to 200 mcg once a day.*	Do not exceed the recommended dosage range unless taking under the direction of a physician.
Tyrosine	500 to 1,000 mg once a day.*	Do not take if you are on an MAO inhibitor antidepressant. Do not take if you have kidney disease unless you are working with a physician. Side effects may include hypertension, hypotension, and migraine headaches.
Vitamin A and mixed carotenoids	5,000 IU—half vitamin A and half mixed carotenoids—once a day.	Use caution when taking vitamin A supplements because they have the potential to be toxic. Do not take high doses if you have liver disease, are a smoker, or have been exposed to asbestos.
Vitamin E	100 to 400 IU a day.*	Do not take with ferrous sulfate iron supplements, which destroy vitamin E. Do not take if you are on a blood-thinning medication. Take mixed tocopherols, the more active type of vitamin E.

| Zinc | 25 mg once a day. | The best-absorbed zinc supplements are zinc picolinate and zinc citrate. Side effects of zinc supplements may include nausea, stomach upset, and heartburn. If these effects persist or worsen, notify your doctor promptly. |

*To choose an appropriate dose, see page 199 for information on dosage ranges.
†See page 197 for information on pharmaceutical-grade supplements.

Most likely, you will have to take some form of thyroid hormone replacement drug, but supplements that raise your T3 levels may help decrease the dosage of this medication. If you have symptoms of gut dysfunction, tell your doctor before starting thyroid medication, as a poorly functioning gut will not be able to absorb it properly. Take advantage of the many ways in which you can improve your thyroid function, but always talk to your doctor before starting any supplement plan alongside traditional drug therapy.

CONCLUSION

While it is never easy to hear that your body isn't working properly, you must speak to your health-care provider if you suspect that you have a thyroid problem. Left unchecked, thyroid hormone dysfunction can lead not only to weight gain but also to a host of other very serious health conditions. But it is very treatable. Hormone replacements and other supplements can put your body back in balance, which, in turn, can help you get rid of added pounds.

Thyroid hormone dysfunction, however, may be just one of several conditions that are contributing to your weight problem. If you still find it difficult to trim your waistline even after you've gotten your thyroid hormones under control, be sure to investigate the other chapters in this book, each of which deals with a different health condition, lifestyle issue, or biochemical factor that may also be preventing you from slimming down. Once you have identified the contributing factors, turn to Chapter 20, "Putting It All Together," which will help you create an integrated weight-loss program that is suited to your needs.

11

Toxic Buildup

You have probably read about the dangers of toxins. Found in the air you breathe, the food you eat, the water you drink, and even in household and personal care products, these poisons can lead to a range of health disorders. But did you know that they can also lead to weight gain?

Toxic buildup may be one of the most overlooked reasons behind the inability to lose weight. While environmental toxins are being linked to more and more diseases every day, they are rarely mentioned in connection with weight gain and loss. A number of chemical pollutants, however, can slowly alter your body's capacity to function properly, affecting your ability to burn calories and shed pounds.

In order to remain healthy and achieve weight loss, your body must detoxify itself through the kidneys, the liver, the skin, and the gastrointestinal tract. Each of these organs, however, can itself be damaged by toxins through environmental exposure, diet, and lifestyle. Once their effectiveness is diminished, a vicious circle begins, often leading to obesity and a host of other illnesses.

Although toxic buildup may seem unavoidable, there are many ways to combat the problem. Once you understand how to identify toxic buildup, you can adjust your diet and lifestyle to eliminate the toxins from your body, and finally get rid of that extra weight.

WHAT IS TOXIC BUILDUP?

A *toxin* can be described as any substance that produces a harmful effect on the body. Whether you are aware of it or not, you are exposed to numerous toxins on a routine basis. Pesticides used in modern farming, industrial chemicals, medications, and other synthetic compounds make

their way into your system every day. According to the Environmental
Protection Agency, more than 4 billion pounds of chemicals were released
into the ground in the year 2000, threatening our natural ground water
sources. Every year, over 2.5 billion pounds of pesticides are dumped on
crop lands, forests, lawns, and fields, while the average American
unknowingly eats about 124 pounds of food additives. Over time, these
compounds can overburden your body's natural detoxifying agents and
build up to unhealthy levels. They can then damage your organs, making
it even more difficult for your body to detoxify itself. While there is simply not enough room in this book to list the thousands of toxins out there,
there are a handful of common environmental poisons of which you
should be aware, including:

- **Asbestos.** Used to insulate ceiling, floors, water pipes, and heating
  ducts until it was banned in the 1970s, asbestos can still be found in
  older homes. It has been linked with scarring of the lung tissue, lung
  cancer, and a rare form of cancer called mesothelioma.

- **Chlorine.** Chlorine is used in household cleaners and to purify drinking water. At unsafe levels, however, it can cause respiratory problems,
  as well as skin and eye irritation.

- **Dioxins.** Dioxins are a family of chemical pollutants that are produced
  by industrial manufacturing. As they are easily stored in fat, they generally make their way into your body through the consumption of meat
  and dairy products. Exposure to high levels of these toxins can result
  in skin lesions, impaired immune function, and cancer.

- **Heavy Metals.** Found in drinking water, fish, pesticides, building
  materials, and even antiperspirants, heavy metals such as mercury,
  lead, and aluminum can cause a variety of health conditions, from
  fatigue and nausea to kidney disease and cancer.

- **PCBs.** Although they have been banned from most uses since 1979,
  polychlorinated biphenyls, or PCBs, remain in the environment, leach-
  ing into water and soil. In particular, these toxins are found in high
  amounts in farm-raised salmon, which ingest PCBs through fish meal.

- **Pesticides.** Still widely used in agriculture, these pest-killing chemicals
  have been linked to cancer, Parkinson's disease, nerve damage, birth
  defects, and miscarriage.

- **Phthalates.** Phthalates are a class of industrial chemical most commonly used in the production of soft plastics and fragrances. They have been linked to the disruption of proper sex hormone function, especially in developing children and fetuses.

- **VOCs.** From paints and varnishes to office equipment and home furnishings, hundreds of everyday products give off volatile organic compounds, or VOCs, in the form of gas. These chemicals have been associated with headaches, eye irritation, memory impairment, and even cancer.

As you can see, toxins seem to be a part of almost every aspect of modern living. Because these poisons cannot be completely avoided, the accumulation of toxins in your system is a very real possibility. This buildup promotes weight gain and can also lead to other serious diseases. It is therefore important to recognize its symptoms.

WHAT ARE THE SYMPTOMS OF TOXIC BUILDUP?

There are a wide variety of symptoms of toxic buildup that can appear throughout your body. They can range from physical discomforts such as bloating and cramps to psychological issues such as confusion and a loss of concentration. Because toxic buildup affects the health of your immune system, some of its symptoms start in your gut, which plays a prominent role not only in fighting disease but also in your metabolism.

With its delicate balance of both healthful and harmful bacteria, the gastrointestinal tract—more commonly known as your gut—has a tremendous influence on your well-being. Toxic buildup often disrupts that balance, leading to a range of possible symptoms, which include:

- Abdominal bloating
- Abdominal pain
- Altered bowel function (constipation or diarrhea)
- Belching
- Cramping
- Flatulence (gas)
- Halitosis (bad breath)
- Heartburn
- Nausea
- Stomach cramps and spasms
- Weight gain

There are also symptoms of toxic buildup that may occur outside of the gastrointestinal tract, including:

- Anxiety
- Confusion
- Depression
- Fatigue
- Fever
- Frequent urination
- General feelings of discomfort or fatigue
- Headaches
- Itching

- Joint pain
- Loss of concentration
- Muscle aches
- Palpitations
- Phlebitis (inflammation of the veins)
- Seizures
- Skin rashes
- Vasculitis (inflammation of the blood vessels)

While these conditions do not always mean that you are suffering from toxic buildup, if several of these symptoms sound familiar to you, perhaps toxic buildup is contributing to your weight-loss problem.

HOW DOES TOXIC BUILDUP CONTRIBUTE TO WEIGHT GAIN?

Pesticides and other toxins have been linked to weight gain, which they contribute to in a number of indirect ways. For example, environmental toxins can sometimes mimic the hormone estrogen in both women and men. Elevated levels of estrogen impair metabolism, increasing fat cells and enhancing the ability of those cells to store fat. (For more information about estrogen, see Chapters 14 and 17.) High amounts of estrogen can also lower thyroid function, which can ultimately result in weight gain (see Chapter 10).

In addition to estrogen-mimicking toxins, other types of chemical pollutants can accumulate in your body, causing inflammation (see Chapter 9), provoking the release of stress hormones such as cortisol (see Chapter 6), and promoting insulin resistance (see Chapter 16), all of which contributes to excess weight. And, unfortunately, these issues do not solely affect adults. The substances absorbed by a pregnant woman can affect her unborn child for years to come. Chemicals such as phthalates and bisphenol A, found in certain plastics and the lining of metal cans, as well as the numerous additives in cigarettes can disrupt the proper hormonal development of a fetus, possibly contributing to childhood obesity.

HOW DO YOU DETERMINE IF YOU HAVE TOXIC BUILDUP?

Stool and urine tests are generally the first method used to check for any toxins or impurities that might be building up in your system. For example, your doctor may order a comprehensive digestive stool diagnosis (CDSA) or GI effects test to determine the health of your bowel, or may perform a pancreatic elastase test, which tests your gut for levels of certain necessary enzymes.

Sometimes toxic buildup is simply a result of genetics, which can cause a poorly functioning detoxification system. Your doctor can order genetic testing, or, in some cases, you can directly order it from one of the laboratories listed on pages 207 to 209 of the "Resources" section. (For more information on genetic testing, see page 149 of Chapter 15.) These tests can determine whether your detoxification organs are working properly and identify potential genetic trouble spots in your self-defense system. Once these trouble spots have been discovered, a physician who specializes in metabolic and anti-aging medicine can design precise individualized therapy to improve your body's ability to convert and expel toxins. (See page 211 for organizations that can guide you to an appropriate health-care provider in your area.)

WHAT CAN YOU DO TO LOSE WEIGHT?

The best way to treat toxic buildup is to avoid exposure to toxins and help your body eliminate the toxins that are already in your system. The following guidelines should help you steer clear of these environmental poisons.

- Avoid the chronic use of medication unless absolutely necessary

- Buy organic produce

- Do not take recreational drugs

- Drink plenty of filtered tap water or spring water

- Eat a diet low in processed foods and fat

- Exercise

- Lessen your occupational exposure to toxins

- Limit your consumption of alcohol

- Quit smoking

- Reduce your consumption of caffeine

- Steer clear of industrial plants and areas of high vehicle traffic

- Wear protective gear when using pesticides, paint, and other toxic substances

Because it is impossible to completely avoid exposure to toxins, you want to keep every aspect of your detoxification system working properly. The key is to provide your detoxifying organs—particularly your liver—with the vitamins, minerals, and other substances they need for optimal performance. The enzymes used by your organs during detoxification are fueled by specific nutrients. Without them, your body may be unable to eliminate toxins. The table below details the compounds that support the detoxification process.

SUPPLEMENTS TO SUPPORT YOUR DETOXIFICATION SYSTEM

Supplement	Dosage	Considerations
B-complex vitamins	Choose a B-complex vitamin that provides 10 to 50 mg each of vitamins B_1, B_2, B_3, B_5, and B_6; 200 to 400 mcg of folic acid; and 250 to 500 mcg of B_{12}. Take twice a day.	Speak to your health-care provider before taking if you have diabetes, liver problems, or anemia. B-complex vitamins may interact with certain antibiotics and anti-seizure medications. Whenever taking a B-complex vitamin, always take a multivitamin as well.
Choline	200 to 250 mg twice a day.	Do not take more than 3 g a day.
Copper	1 to 3 mg once a day.*	Your copper-to-zinc ratio is very important for your health. Always take zinc if you are taking copper. Do not take copper if you have Wilson's disease. Also do not take the copper supplement cupric oxide, which has a very low bioavailability.
Glutamine	5 to 10 g once a day.*	If you are sensitive to monosodium glutamate (MSG), use glutamine with caution, as your body metabolizes it into glutamate. If you are taking anti-seizure medication, use glutamine only under the direction of your doctor.

Glycine	250 to 1,500 mg twice a day.*	Do not take glycine if you are taking clozapine or another atypical antipsychotic medication.
Magnesium	400 to 800 mg once a day.*	Consult health-care provider for dosage if you have kidney disease. Discontinue use and see your doctor if you experience abdominal pain. Take a lower dose if it causes diarrhea. Magnesium's citrate, glycinate, gluconate, and lactate forms are more easily absorbed than its oxide form.
Methionine	250 mg once a day.	High levels can reduce the effectiveness of levodopa, a drug used to treat Parkinson's disease.
Molybdenum	75 to 250 mcg once a day.*	Large doses of 10 to 15 mg a day can cause your body to lose copper and have been associated with gout-like symptoms such as warmth, pain, swelling, and extreme tenderness in a joint (usually the big toe).
Multivitamin, pharmaceutical-grade†	Follow the directions on the bottle.	Make sure to take only a pharmaceutical-grade multivitamin.
N-acetylcysteine (NAC)	250 to 1,500 mg twice a day.*	NAC can cause kidney stones, which can be avoided by taking 500 to 1,000 mg of vitamin C once a day. You may also need to take extra copper and zinc, as NAC reduces the effectiveness of these elements. Speak to your doctor about monitoring blood levels of these minerals.
S-adenosyl-methionine (SAMe)	200 to 400 mg twice a day.*	Do not take if you have a bipolar disorder.
Taurine	500 to 1,000 mg once a day.*	Take between meals. Do not take with aspirin or any salicylate. Check with your health-care provider before taking taurine if you have kidney disease. Discontinue use if you suddenly have feelings of chest or throat tightness or if you break out in hives.
Trimethylglycine (TMG)	400 to 500 mg twice a day.	Side effects may include dry mouth, headache, diarrhea, nausea, and upset stomach.

| Vitamin C | 1,000 mg once a day. | Doses higher than 5,000 mg may cause diarrhea. Mineral ascorbates and Ester-C are buffered forms of vitamin C that lower the chance of diarrhea. Do not take high doses if you are prone to kidney stones or gout. |
| Zinc | 25 mg once a day. | The best-absorbed zinc supplements are zinc picolinate and zinc citrate. Side effects of zinc supplements may include nausea, stomach upset, and heartburn. If these effects persist or worsen, notify your doctor promptly. |

*To choose an appropriate dose, see page 199 for information on dosage ranges.
† See page 197 for information on pharmaceutical-grade supplements.

Once your body has begun to detoxify itself, you should take steps to restore health to your gut. Start the healing process by eating high-fiber foods, such as okra and cabbage. In addition, repopulate your gastrointestinal system with healthful bacteria by eating fermented foods such as yogurt. Finally, use aloe vera, glutamine, and licorice root—all listed in the table below—to repair your small bowel, heal your large bowel, and promote good gastrointestinal function.

SUPPLEMENTS TO REPAIR GASTROINTESTINAL FUNCTION

Supplement	Dosage	Considerations
Aloe vera	Up to 150 mg once a day.	When taken orally, aloe vera can cause diarrhea and nausea. Abuse of aloe vera can result in electrolyte imbalances, including low potassium.
Glutamine	5 to 10 g once a day.*	If you have a sensitivity to monosodium glutamate (MSG), use glutamine with caution, as your body metabolizes glutamine into glutamate. If you are taking medications for seizures, use glutamine only under the direction of your doctor.
Licorice root (*Glycyrrhiza glabra*)	600 mg twice a day.	Consult your physician before taking if you have high blood pressure; glaucoma; diabetes; or heart, kidney, or liver disease.

*To choose an appropriate dose, see page 199 for information on dosage ranges.

Simply put, healthy organs make it easier for your body to detoxify itself. Once your body is free of toxic buildup, you should be more able to lose weight and keep it off.

CONCLUSION

If you have been consistently trying to lose weight without seeing any results, your body's toxic burden may be at fault. Pollutants can affect your body's ability to cleanse itself of impurities, which can then build up in your system, causing a range of symptoms and disorders that contribute to weight gain and make it harder to lose added pounds. By reducing your exposure to toxins and providing your body with the vitamins, minerals, and other compounds it needs to cleanse itself of poisonous substances, you can finally make a dent in your waistline.

Toxic buildup, however, may not be the only obstacle standing between you and your ideal weight. If you take steps to detoxify your system and still don't see a change in the number on your scale, be sure to explore the other chapters in this book, each of which examines a specific lifestyle issue, health problem, or biochemical factor that may be affecting your efforts to reduce. Once you have identified the contributing factors, turn to Chapter 20, "Putting It All Together," which will help you create an integrated weight-loss program that is suited to your needs.

12

Yeast Infection

Most women have a vaginal yeast infection at some time in their lives. Usually, this infection is easy to identify and, with the use of medication, almost as easy to treat. But yeast infections—often referred to as *candidiasis*, because the candida species is the most common cause—don't always limit themselves to one area of the body and don't always announce themselves through readily identified symptoms. Under certain circumstances, the yeast organism can multiply and spread uncontrolled. This can result in chronic infections that lead to a wide range of health problems, including weight gain and difficulty in losing excess pounds. To make matters worse, because the symptoms of candidiasis can be so varied, physicians often fail to recognize the underlying difficulty and treat it appropriately. And by the time a widespread infection is discovered, the yeast—which penetrates and damages the body's cells—may be difficult to eliminate.

Although this scenario might sound frightening, the truth is that no one has to suffer with yeast infections. Laboratory tests can determine whether you have yeast overgrowth, and a multileveled treatment plan can spell the end of candidiasis, restoring your well-being and enabling you to enjoy a healthy body weight.

WHAT ARE YEAST INFECTIONS?

The yeast candida is one of the billions of microorganisms normally found in the mucous membranes of the body—in the mouth, the throat, the digestive tract, and the genitals. When the body is working properly, growth of this organism is controlled by the body's healthy bacteria, but when the body's microorganisms get out of balance—which can happen for a number of reasons—yeast can multiply and cause the infection known as *candidiasis*. Most people have heard of vaginal yeast infections; in fact, over one million women in the United States alone develop this disorder every year. Localized infections can also occur in the mouth, where the problem is known as *thrush*, and in other areas of the body, such as the urinary tract. In rare cases, yeast can enter the bloodstream and spread throughout the body, producing a serious systemic infection that can affect the blood, esophagus, eyes, heart, kidneys, liver, skin, and spleen. Infections can and do occur in men as well as women.

There are many factors that can lead to yeast overgrowth, with antibiotics being the leading cause. When these drugs are used to kill disease-causing bacteria, they also destroy the "good" bacteria that keeps yeast and other microorganisms under control. As a result, the yeast is able to multiply and "take over" the body. But antibiotics are not the only cause of yeast infection. The overgrowth of yeast can be set off by just about anything that disturbs the body's delicate balance of microorganisms or compromises the immune system. Possible causes and contributing factors can include the following:

- AIDS
- Alcohol
- Antacids
- Antibiotics
- Birth control pills
- Chemotherapy
- Chronic constipation or diarrhea
- Diabetes
- Excessive stress
- Exposure to chemicals and toxins
- Genital irritations and abrasions
- High blood sugar levels
- Hormonal changes associated with the normal menstrual cycle
- Hypothyroidism (thyroid hormone deficiency)
- Infection from sexual partner
- Intestinal parasites
- Pregnancy
- Steroids

WHAT ARE THE SYMPTOMS OF YEAST INFECTION?

You have already learned that yeast infections can remain very local or can spread throughout the body and affect more than one body system.

The Different Species of Candida Yeast

Often, health professionals specifically refer to *Candida albicans* when discussing yeast infections. It's true that this species is the most common of the candida yeast and, therefore, the most likely culprit when people develop yeast-related disorders. However, there are actually six different species of candida that are responsible for infections in humans.

- *Candida albicans* is the most abundant species of candida and the most frequent cause of vaginal candidiasis. It is believed to be responsible for 50 percent of other candida infections, as well.

- *Candida tropicalis* is the second most common yeast organism to cause infections in humans. It is estimated to be involved in 15 to 30 percent of blood infections from yeast.

- *Candida glabrata* is a common cause of oral yeast infections, and is believed to be involved in 15 to 30 percent of all infections from yeast.

- *Candida parapsilosis* is a species on the rise, and is estimated to cause 15 to 30 percent of all yeast infections.

- *Candida krusei* is a fairly rare species of yeast, accounting for perhaps 1 percent of candidiasis cases. It is most often associated with infant diarrhea and, on occasion, with systemic yeast infections.

- *Candida lusitaniae* is another rare species of candida. It is believed to be responsible for about 1 percent of all candida infections.

For this reason, there is a wide range of possible symptoms of candidiasis. Below, you will find these warning signs categorized according to the area of the body that is affected by the yeast.

Allergic and Upper Respiratory Symptoms

- Asthma
- Blurred vision
- Body aches and tension
- Bronchitis (recurrent)
- Burning or tingling of the extremities
- Chemical sensitivity
- Chest pain
- Coughing
- Earache
- Hay fever

- Headache
- Hives
- Nasal congestion
- Numbness of the extremities
- Painful, swollen, stiff joints
- Shortness of breath
- Sinusitis (sinus infection)
- Sore throat

Cognitive Problems

- Attention deficit hyperactivity disorder (ADD/ADHD)
- Confusion
- Disorientation
- Drowsiness
- Fatigue
- Feelings of unreality
- Hyperactivity
- Inability to concentrate
- Poor memory

Emotional Problems

- Anxiety
- Depression
- Irritability
- Mood swings
- Nervousness
- Obsessive-compulsive disorder

Gastrointestinal Problems

- Bloating
- Constipation
- Crohn's disease
- Diarrhea
- Dry mouth
- Food sensitivities
- Gas
- Halitosis (bad breath)
- Heartburn
- Indigestion
- Inflammation
- Irritable bowel syndrome (IBS)
- Lactose intolerance
- Oral thrush
- Rectal itching

Genital and Reproductive Problems

- Endometriosis
- Impotency
- Infertility
- Loss of sexual feelings

- Menstrual irregularities
- Painful intercourse
- Penile burning, itching, discharge, or rash
- Premenstrual syndrome (PMS)
- Prostatitis (inflammation of the prostate gland)

- Recurrent vaginitis (inflammation of the vagina)
- Uterine cramps
- Vaginal burning, itching, or discharge
- Vulvodynia (chronic vulvar pain)

Glandular and Autoimmune Problems

- Adrenal dysfunction
- Cold hands or feet
- Diabetes
- Hypoglycemia (low blood sugar)
- Hypothyroidism (thyroid hormone deficiency)

- Low body temperature
- Lupus erythematosus
- Multiple sclerosis
- Rheumatoid arthritis
- Scleroderma

Skin Problems

- Acne
- Athlete's foot
- Dandruff
- Diaper rash
- Dry skin
- Eczema
- Excessive perspiration

- Facial rash
- Fungus infection of the nails
- Impetigo (skin infection)
- Inflammation of hair follicles
- Psoriasis
- Seborrheic dermatitis
- Tinea cruris (jock itch)

Urinary Problems

- Bladder infection (recurrent)
- Burning on urination
- Cystitis (inflammation of the bladder)

- Fluid retention
- Frequent urination

Other Disorders

- Chronic fatigue syndrome
- Fibromyalgia
- Insomnia

- Muscle aches or weakness
- Myasthenia gravis

If several of the symptoms in the above lists sound familiar to you, perhaps yeast infection is contributing to your weight-loss problem.

HOW DO YEAST INFECTIONS CONTRIBUTE TO WEIGHT GAIN?

The chief way in which the overgrowth of yeast can increase body weight is by causing you to eat excessive amounts of certain unhealthy foods. When yeast is out of control, it has a hunger all its own: To survive, it needs simple carbohydrates such as those found in flour, sugar, pasta, cake, and ice cream. As strange as it may seem, the yeast actually causes you to have cravings for these high-calorie, nutritionally poor foods. Over time, a vicious cycle develops. The yeast makes you eat more carbs, the carbs fuel the multiplication and spread of the yeast, and the growing colonies of yeast demand even more high-carb treats, leading to the further accumulation of body fat.

As yeast takes over the body, it can also cause added pounds in indirect ways. If you've read the potential symptoms of yeast infection listed on pages 103 through 106, you know that this health problem can cause anxiety, depression, fatigue, and hypothyroidism. All of these disorders can lead to unwanted pounds, either by causing overeating or by slowing your metabolism. (For more information on these conditions and their relationship to weight gain, see Chapters 6, 13, 5, and 10, respectively.) Yeast is also a chief cause of gas, constipation, and bloating, which can make you look and feel heavier than you really are.

HOW DO YOU DETERMINE IF YOU HAVE
A CHRONIC YEAST INFECTION?

An occasional short-term yeast infection should not cause chronic health problems such as excessive weight gain, but if you suspect that your health is being compromised by a long-term yeast infection, your doctor can perform tests to check for yeast overgrowth. Your doctor may ask for a stool (feces) sample, which can be studied under a microscope to reveal the presence of candida in the digestive system. If there is evidence of thrush, an oral yeast infection, your doctor may also choose to swab the inside of your mouth and culture the sample for candida. Another way to determine if there is an overgrowth of candida is the blood analysis known as the Candida Immune Complex Assay. This test can confirm the presence of antibodies that are produced by the body's immune system to combat yeast.

WHAT CAN YOU DO TO LOSE WEIGHT?

If tests have determined that you have a chronic yeast infection, you can regain your health and help lose unwanted weight by taking steps to eliminate yeast from your body. Conventional medical treatment usually includes a prescription antifungal agent, such as nystatin (Mycostatin) or fluconazol (Diflucan). During drug therapy, it can be quite helpful to modify your diet to eliminate sugar and high-sugar foods, processed foods, and any foods that may contain fungi or mold. In particular, you should avoid the following:

- Alcohol
- Breads, pastries, and all yeast-raised bakery goods
- Cheeses
- Condiments, sauces, and vinegars
- Dried and candied fruits
- Edible fungi (mushrooms, morels, and truffles)
- Leftovers
- Malt products
- Melons
- Processed and smoked meats

You can further speed your recovery from yeast infection by taking probiotics (health-promoting bacteria) as well as the other nutritional supplements listed in the table "Supplements to Treat Candidiasis," found on page 108.

SUPPLEMENTS TO TREAT CANDIDIASIS

Supplement	Dosage	Considerations
Berberine sulfate hydrate	100 mg once a day.	Do not take if you are pregnant or breastfeeding.
Caprylic acid	600 mg once a day.	Do not take if you are pregnant or nursing. Can cause nausea, bloating, constipation, or diarrhea.
Cinnamon bark extract	100 mg once a day.	Cinnamon can lower your blood sugar. If you are taking a medication for blood sugar control, check your blood sugar levels and make adjustments as necessary. A lower dosage of medication may be needed.
Copper	1 to 3 mg once a day.*	Your copper-to-zinc ratio is very important for your health. Always take zinc if you are taking copper. Do not take copper if you have Wilson's disease. Also, do not take the copper supplement cupric oxide, which has a very low bioavailability.
Garlic (*Allium sativum*)	400 mg twice a day.	Do not take if you are on a blood-thinning medication.
Ginger root (*Zingiber officinale*)	500 mg twice a day.	Do not take if you are on a blood-thinning medication or NSAIDs. If you have allergies, cardiac problems, central nervous system problems, or renal problems, consult with your health-care provider before taking ginger.
Glutamine	5 to 10 g once a day.*	If you have a sensitivity to monosodium glutamate (MSG), use glutamine with caution, as your body metabolizes glutamine into glutamate. If you are taking medications for seizures, use glutamine only under the direction of your doctor.
Grapefruit seed extract	125 mg once a day.	Do not take if you are allergic to citrus fruits.
Multivitamin, pharmaceutical-grade†	Follow the directions on the bottle.	Make sure to take only a pharmaceutical-grade multivitamin.
Olive leaf extract	500 mg twice a day.	Take with food.
Oregano leaf extract	100 mg once a day.	Do not take if you are allergic to the Lamiaceae family of plants, which includes basil, hyssop, lavender, marjoram, mint, and sage.

Oregon grape root	70 to 100 mg once a day.	Do not take if you are pregnant.
Pau d'Arco inner bark extract	100 mg once a day.	Do not take if you are on a blood-thinning medication.
Probiotics	20 billion units once a day.	If using an antibiotic, wait three hours before taking probiotics.
Rosemary leaf extract	100 mg once a day.	Do not take if you have iron deficiency anemia.
Taurine	500 to 1,000 mg once a day.*	Take between meals. Do not take with aspirin or any salicylate. Check with your health-care provider before taking taurine if you have kidney disease. Discontinue use if you suddenly have feelings of chest or throat tightness or if you break out in hives.
Undecylenic acid	200 mg three times a day.	If you are pregnant or breastfeeding, discuss with your doctor before using.
Zinc	25 mg once a day.	The best-absorbed zinc supplements are zinc picolinate and zinc citrate. Side effects of zinc supplements may include nausea, stomach upset, and heartburn. If these effects persist or worsen, notify your doctor promptly.

*To choose an appropriate dose, see page 199 for information on dosage ranges.
†See page 197 for information on pharmaceutical-grade supplements.

CONCLUSION

If a long-term yeast infection is keeping you from shedding pounds, there is much you can do to improve your health. The proper medication, smart dietary restrictions, and appropriate nutritional supplementation can eliminate yeast from your system and help you reach the desired weight.

On the other hand, an overgrowth of yeast may be just one of several factors that are keeping you from looking and feeling your best. If you take steps to treat this disorder and are still unable to lose weight, be sure to explore the other chapters in this book, each of which examines a specific lifestyle issue, health problem, or biochemical factor that may be affecting your efforts to reduce. Once you have identified the contributing factors, turn to Chapter 20, "Putting It All Together," which will help you create an integrated weight-loss program that is suited to your needs.

PART III

Biochemical Factors

Introduction
to Part III

Your body is a sophisticated machine that, in order to function, must produce and react to literally thousands of chemicals. Most of the time, you remain happily unaware of these substances. You're healthy, and all those biochemicals—estrogen, insulin, and serotonin, to name just a few—do their job without your giving them a thought. But sometimes, one or more substances are produced in the wrong amounts or your body simply stops responding to them as it should. When this happens, you can experience a range of symptoms and problems, including excess weight and difficulty in shedding pounds.

Part III focuses on biochemistry-related disorders that have been linked to excess weight. Depression and its treatment, female hormone imbalance, insulin resistance, male hormone deficiency, neurotransmitter dysfunction, and pregnenolone insufficiency can all lead to weight gain and make it difficult to lose unwanted pounds. You may even have a genetic predisposition that causes you to gain weight. In each chapter, you'll learn about the biochemical issue being examined, read about its symptoms, and discover how it can lead to weight gain. You will then find guidelines—including, in some cases, laboratory tests—for determining if this problem is affecting your health. Finally, you'll discover the many ways in which you can begin treatment, using diet, exercise, nutritional supplements, and more, so that your body can recover its biochemical balance and reach a healthy weight.

If you feel that an underlying problem may be hampering your efforts to shed excess pounds, take the self-test presented on page 113. If your answers indicate that biochemical issues may be involved, Chapters 13 through 19 will guide you in taking important steps towards a healthier, slimmer body.

BIOCHEMICAL FACTOR QUESTIONNAIRE

This test was designed to help you determine if biochemical factors, such as hormone dysfunction, may be hindering your attempts to lose weight. For each of the following questions, check the box that most accurately applies to you. When you have completed the questionnaire, count the number of times you answered "Often." If you checked this answer more than ten times, chances are that one or more disorders are compromising your ability to lose unwanted pounds. Read Chapters 13 through 19 to learn why your answers may indicate a problem, and how treating biochemical-related disorders can make it easier to lose weight.

	Seldom	Sometimes	Often
1. Do you have trouble concentrating on tasks?	☐	☐	☐
2. Do you have trouble remembering things?	☐	☐	☐
3. Do you find yourself frustrated by even minor problems?	☐	☐	☐
4. Do you experience confusion?	☐	☐	☐
5. Do you experience extreme sadness or melancholy?	☐	☐	☐
6. Do you feel anxious and irritable?	☐	☐	☐
7. Do you experience mood swings?	☐	☐	☐
8. Do you prefer staying home to engaging in social activities?	☐	☐	☐
9. Do you have cravings for sweet and/or salty foods?	☐	☐	☐
10. Do you have trouble losing weight even when you stick to a weight-loss diet?	☐	☐	☐
11. Do you feel tired immediately after eating a meal?	☐	☐	☐

	Seldom	Sometimes	Often
12. Do you have inappropriate hunger, such as hunger after eating a large meal?	☐	☐	☐
13. Do you experience loose bowel movements alternating with constipation?	☐	☐	☐
14. Do you suffer from backache, stiffness, or joint pain?	☐	☐	☐
15. Do you experience headaches and migraines?	☐	☐	☐
16. Do you experience fluid retention and bloating?	☐	☐	☐
17. Do you have trouble falling or staying asleep?	☐	☐	☐
18. Do you experience hot flashes and/or night sweats?	☐	☐	☐
19. Do you feel a decrease in sexual interest?	☐	☐	☐
20. Do you experience erectile dysfunction (inability to develop or maintain an erection)?	☐	☐	☐
TOTALS	_____	_____	_____

13

Depression and Antidepressants

For weeks, you've been feeling terrible—not sick exactly, but sad and hopeless. Nothing really happened to make you feel this way, and your friends are urging you to "snap out of it." But you can't snap out of it; you can barely summon the will to get out of bed in the morning. All the things you had planned to do—like finally going on that diet—have fallen by the wayside. In fact, you seem to be gaining more weight rather than taking it off. What's going on?

In the United States alone, more than 17 million people are estimated to suffer with depression in any given year, and the condition is common throughout the world. In fact, this illness has been called the "common cold" of mental health disorders. In its mildest form, depression causes feelings of unhappiness and a loss of interest in everyday activities. When it persists for a long period of time, it can lead to physical changes that increase the risk of type 2 diabetes and cardiovascular disease. At its worst, it can result in self-inflicted harm.

Health experts know that weight gain and depression often go hand in hand. Although researchers aren't absolutely sure of the process through which this mental health problem leads to excess pounds, they have long observed that people who suffer from depression and other mental disorders are more likely than others to gain weight and become obese over time. In addition, there is the well-known connection between antidepressants and weight gain. Prescription medications are often successful in helping people manage depression, but they cause weight gain in 25 percent of the people who take them, especially when the drugs are used over the long-term.

Fortunately, there is much that can be done to alleviate depression. The first important step is to understand what it is and how it can be identified. You can then take important steps to ease depression and resolve the very real physical problems it can cause.

WHAT IS DEPRESSION?

Depression is a medical disorder that involves both the mind and the body. Far more than a case of the blues, it is a feeling of unhappiness, melancholy, or despair that lasts for a prolonged period of time—weeks, months, or even years. It often recurs over time, requiring long-term care, just like diabetes or heart disease.

Although depression is sometimes thought of as being extreme sadness, there is big difference between sadness and *clinical depression,* which is also called *chronic depression, major depression,* and *major depressive disorder.* Everyone experiences sadness at some time in their lives, usually as the result of unpleasant circumstances, such as the loss of a job or the death of a loved one. In time, the sadness lifts as the individual deals with life's problems. But in the case of clinical depression, the feelings last much longer and the individual often doesn't know their cause. Furthermore, while people who are sad usually manage to cope with living and perform everyday activities, those who are clinically depressed may feel overwhelmed and unable to deal with life. Moreover, depression usually includes many symptoms that are not associated with a temporary case of the blues.

WHAT ARE THE SYMPTOMS OF DEPRESSION?

The symptoms of depression can vary from person to person, and also according to age. Below, you will find the signs that are characteristic of adult depression. Following this, you will find symptoms of depression that are specific to certain age groups. Be aware that older adults may also have the common signs of adult depression, but that some of these problems—fatigue, loss of appetite, and reduced interest in sex, for instance—typically go unrecognized because they are seen as being part of aging or of another illness. It's important to recognize *all* behaviors and feelings while determining if you or someone you know is suffering from depression.

Common Symptoms of Adult Depression

- Agitation or restlessness, resulting in hand-wringing or pacing
- Crying spells without cause
- Decreased appetite and weight loss

- Increased appetite and weight gain
- Excessive sleeping
- Fatigue
- Feelings of sadness
- Feelings of worthlessness or guilt
- Frequent thoughts of death or suicide
- Frustration and irritability, even over small events
- Indecisiveness
- Insomnia
- Intense cravings for certain foods
- Loss of concentration
- Loss of interest in activities that are normally pleasurable
- Reduced sex drive
- Slowness in thinking, speaking, or moving
- Unexplained physical problems such as backache

Symptoms Characteristic of Adolescent and Teen Depression

- Anxiety and anger
- Avoidance of social situations
- Behavior and mental health problems such as attention deficit hyperactivity disorder (ADHD)

Symptoms Characteristic of Older Adult Depression

- Desire to stay home
- Feelings of boredom and dissatisfaction with life
- Thoughts of suicide

If several of the symptoms in the above lists sound familiar to you, perhaps depression is contributing to your weight-loss problem.

HOW DOES DEPRESSION CONTRIBUTE TO WEIGHT GAIN?

For a long time, people assumed that gaining excess weight caused people to become depressed—that the weight gain came first and, because of the stigma attached to excess weight, feelings of sadness and hopelessness followed. But several long-term studies have shown that depression, anxiety, and other mental health disorders actually increase weight gain and, in time, often lead to obesity. One British study found that during a nineteen-year period, people who reported at least three episodes of depression or another mental illness were *twice* as likely to become obese as people who reported themselves as happy. The more times an individual reported mental health symptoms, the greater the risk of obesity. An American study found that people with symptoms of depression gain weight more rapidly than people who don't suffer from this disorder, and that this weight gain is most noticeable in the belly.

The reason for this relationship between depression and weight gain is not absolutely clear to researchers, but several factors seem to be at work. First, people who are depressed tend to be inactive, to exercise less, and to eat more than people who do not have mental health problems. The lack of activity combined with overeating leads to weight gain.

Experts also think that depression is often caused by increased stress and, specifically, by an increase in the stress hormone *cortisol*. When cortisol levels rise due to prolonged stress, the body puts on more weight, especially in the abdominal area. In addition, chronically elevated cortisol levels reduce levels of the body's feel-good chemicals, such as dopamine, potentially leading to a state of depression. So chronic stress can simultaneously cause weight gain *and* depression. (To learn more about stress and weight gain, see Chapter 6.)

Of course, in some cases, weight gain may actually lead to mental health problems. Because our society worships thinness and attaches a stigma to excess weight, being obese or even a few pounds overweight can cause you to experience lowered self-esteem, sadness, and eventually, clinical depression. Since depression itself can lead to added pounds, this can make the situation spiral out of control. Obesity and depression are so interrelated that it is difficult to separate the two.

Antidepressants

Most antidepressants have been associated with weight gain in some patients. Studies have shown that the antidepressant bupropion (Wellbutrin) may not cause weight gain, and actually causes weight loss in some people. But the effects of these drugs are very individual. An antidepressant that leads to weight gain in one person may not put on pounds in another individual.

Again, experts are not sure why antidepressants tend to cause weight gain, but it is believed that in different people, weight problems develop for different reasons. Sometimes, the medication is not a direct cause of weight problems. In those people who actually lose interest in eating due to depression, for instance, antidepressants can cause weight gain simply by making the individuals feel better and eat more. But in other people, antidepressants may more directly lead to an increase in weight. All antidepressants appear to work by blocking the brain's response to chemical messengers. Many of these drugs, while alleviating depression, also block the effect of brain chemicals that would normally control body weight. By stopping the activity of these chemicals, the drug can cause a general increase in appetite; cravings for specific foods, such as carbohydrates; or even an increase in weight despite no obvious increase in eating.

HOW DO YOU DETERMINE IF YOU SUFFER FROM DEPRESSION?

According to current medical guidelines, you are suffering from clinical depression if you have been experiencing intense sadness and loss of interest in daily activities for at least a two-week period. This mood must represent a change from your usual frame of mind and must not be the result of a general medical condition or of the use of alcohol or drugs. The symptoms listed on pages 116 to 117 should help you determine if you are suffering the effects of depression.

If you suspect that you are depressed, it is important to visit your family doctor for a complete checkup. There is no current test that can be used to diagnose depression, but a doctor can determine if you have any medical conditions, such as thyroid problems, that can cause depressive symptoms, or if any medication you are taking has depressive side effects. A physician can also evaluate the signs of depression that you have noted on your own, ask you about further symptoms, and examine your medical history. Because depression may not only have a great impact on your life, but, in extreme cases, lead to self-harm, a professional consultation is a vital component of your treatment.

If it is determined that you are clinically depressed, your doctor may suggest therapy as well as a course of medication. The lifestyle changes that are recommended in the following section may help you relieve feelings of depression and, in the process, aid you in losing those unwanted pounds.

WHAT CAN YOU DO TO LOSE WEIGHT?

Inactivity is a common symptom of depression and contributes to the weight gain associated with both this and other mental health disorders. It should come as no surprise, then, that one way you can lose the weight due to depression is to exercise. What may surprise you is that physical activity can actually lighten your mood. Studies have shown that Americans who exercise on a regular basis suffer less depression than those who are inactive, and are also less likely to experience recurrences of depression in the future. In one study, the power of aerobic exercise to boost mood was found equal to that of antidepressants—and caused no side effects. Researchers don't know why this occurs but believe that exercise may actually alter brain activity to reduce the stress response that can lead to depression. Whatever the reason, it seems clear that physical activity can help you fight depression and weight gain while providing all the other health benefits that exercise has to offer. (See Chapter 2 for more information about weight loss and exercise.)

In addition to stepping up your activity level, you can relieve depression by using the appropriate nutritional supplements. Certain nutritional deficiencies are associated with this disorder—deficiencies of the B vitamins, calcium, and copper for instance—so by following a good supplement plan (see the table below), you can improve your mood while boosting your overall health. Just be sure to consult your physician about the nutritional aspect of your treatment, because certain medications (including antidepressants) may contraindicate the use of some nutritional supplements.

SUPPLEMENTS TO TREAT DEPRESSION		
Supplement	Dosage	Considerations
Alpha-lipoic acid	100 mg once a day.	Improves blood sugar levels, so diabetics may be able to take less medication. If you have diabetes and are taking alpha-lipoic acid, check your blood sugar regularly.

Ashwagandha root	500 to 1,000 mg once a day.*	Do not take if you are pregnant. Possible side effects may include nausea, vomiting, and diarrhea.
B-complex vitamins	Choose a B-complex vitamin that provides 10 to 50 mg each of vitamins B_1, B_2, B_3, B_5, and B_6; 200 to 400 mcg of folic acid; and 250 to 500 mcg of B_{12}. Take twice a day.	Speak to your health-care provider before taking if you have diabetes, liver problems, or anemia. B-complex vitamins may interact with certain antibiotics and anti-seizure medications. Whenever taking a B-complex vitamin, always take a multivitamin as well.
Calcium	• 250 to 500 mg once a day for men. • 500 mg once a day for premenopausal women. • 800 mg once a day for perimenopausal women. • 1,000 mg once a day for menopausal women.	Although most people are deficient in calcium, there is a danger in taking too much. Do not ingest more than 1,000 to 1,200 mg of calcium a day.
Chromium	400 mcg once a day.	Combining chromium with the protein picolinate allows your body to absorb the nutrient more efficiently. If you have kidney disease, consult your physician before taking chromium.
Coenzyme Q_{10}	60 to 200 mg once a day. If you are using over 100 mg a day, take in divided doses.*	May reduce the effects of blood-thinning medication. May cause diarrhea in dosages above 100 mg once a day.
Copper	1 to 3 mg once a day.*	Your copper-to-zinc ratio is very important for your health. Always take zinc if you are taking copper. Do not take copper if you have Wilson's disease. Also do not take the copper supplement cupric oxide, which has a very low bioavailability.
5-Hydroxy-tryptophan (5-HTP)	25 to 150 mg twice a day.*	Do not take 5-HTP if you are taking an SSRI, MAO inhibitor, or other antidepressant.
Ginkgo (Ginkgo biloba)	120 mg once a day.	Do not take if you are on a blood-thinning medication.
Ginseng	500 mg once a day	Always take with food. Do not use if you are taking a blood-thinning medication. Use with caution if you have high blood pressure.

L-Carnitine	500 to 1,000 mg once a day.*	Side effects are rare but can include agitation, headache, increased appetite, nausea, skin rashes, and vomiting. Ask your doctor before taking if you have kidney or liver disease.
Magnesium	400 to 800 mg once a day.*	Consult health-care provider for dosage if you have kidney disease. Discontinue use and see your doctor if you experience abdominal pain. Take a lower dose if it causes diarrhea. Magnesium's citrate, glycinate, gluconate, and lactate forms are more easily absorbed than its oxide form.
Multivitamin, pharmaceutical-grade**	Follow the directions on the bottle.	Make sure to take only a pharmaceutical-grade multivitamin.
Omega-3 essential fatty acids EPA/DHA (fish oil)	1,000 to 3,000 mg once a day.*	In dosages above 4,000 mg, may cause the blood to thin. Do not take more than 4,000 mg a day if you are using a blood-thinning medication.
Phosphatidyl-choline	1,000 to 2,000 mg once a day.*	Use with caution if you have malabsorption problems, as this could exacerbate them.
Phosphatidyl-serine	300 mg once a day.	Do not take if you are on a blood-thinning medication. Use with caution if you are also taking medication to treat depression, glaucoma, or Alzheimer's disease. Do not take if you are pregnant or breastfeeding. Side effects may include insomnia and stomach upset.
St. John's Wort (*Hypericum perforatum*)	300 to 400 mg three times a day.*	Do not take with antidepressants, indinavir, cyclosporine, theophylline, warfarin, or ethinylestradiol. If you are exposed to the sun, it may cause a skin rash. May lessen the effects of birth control pills.
Selenium	100 to 200 mcg once a day.*	Do not exceed the recommended dosage range unless taking under the direction of a physician.
Tryptophan, pharmaceutical grade†	Your physician must prescribe the appropriate dosage.	Make sure to take only pharmaceutical-grade tryptophan. Do not take if you are on an antidepressant. Do not take if you have kidney disease unless you are working with a physician.

Tyrosine	500 to 1,000 mg once a day.*	Do not take if you are on an MAO inhibitor antidepressant. Do not take if you have kidney disease unless you are working with a physician. Side effects may include hypertension, hypotension, and migraine headaches.
Vitamin A and mixed carotenoids	5,000 IU—half vitamin A and half mixed carotenoids—once a day.	Use caution when taking vitamin A supplements because they have the potential to be toxic. Do not take high doses if you have liver disease, are a smoker, or have been exposed to asbestos.
Vitamin C	1,000 mg once a day.	Doses higher than 5,000 mg may cause diarrhea. Mineral ascorbates and Ester-C are buffered forms of vitamin C that lower the chance of diarrhea. Do not take high doses if you are prone to kidney stones or gout.
Zinc	25 mg once a day.	The best-absorbed zinc supplements are zinc picolinate and zinc citrate. Side effects of zinc supplements may include nausea, stomach upset, and heartburn. If these effects persist or worsen, notify your doctor promptly.

*To choose an appropriate dose, see page 199 for information on dosage ranges.
†See page 197 for information on pharmaceutical-grade supplements.

Finally, if you feel that your weight gain has been caused or worsened by the use of an antidepressant, speak to your doctor about switching to another medication. As discussed on page 119, some of these drugs are more likely than others to cause weight gain, and while one antidepressant may cause you to put on pounds, another might not.

CONCLUSION

If depression is preventing you from shedding pounds, there is a lot you can do to improve your mood and eliminate depressive symptoms. In many cases, exercise and appropriate nutritional supplementation can treat this condition, enhance your overall health, and help you reach your desired weight.

On the other hand, depression may be just one of several factors that are keeping you from shedding pounds. If you take steps to treat this disorder and still are unable to lose weight, be sure to explore the other chapters in this book, each of which examines a specific lifestyle issue, health problem, or biochemical factor that may be affecting your efforts to reduce. Once you have identified the contributing factors, turn to Chapter 20, "Putting It All Together," which will help you create an integrated weight-loss program that is suited to your needs.

14

Female Hormonal Imbalance

Every woman knows that hormones play a vital role in the function of the body. When they are produced in the proper amounts and are in balance with one another, you feel healthy and look great. When they are not, a number of health problems can occur. Weight gain is one of them.

This chapter examines female hormones and their roles in three common hormonal conditions—premenstrual syndrome (PMS), polycystic ovarian syndrome (PCOS), and perimenopause/menopause. Each condition has a direct influence on a woman's body weight. First we will take a look at the main female sex hormones—what they are, what overall functions they perform, and what problems are associated with their imbalance. Next, we will examine the three conditions influenced by these hormones as they relate to weight gain.

WHAT ARE THE FEMALE SEX HORMONES?

Estrogen, progesterone, and testosterone are among the female sex hormones that are influential in weight gain. They play important roles in manipulating metabolism, determining how fat is stored, and controlling food cravings. As you will see, when these hormones are out of balance or not produced in sufficient amounts, excess weight and a range of other unpleasant side effects and health conditions may result.

Estrogen

The most well-known of the traditionally "female" hormones, estrogen is produced primarily in the ovaries. Estrogen has over 400 crucial functions in your body. It is responsible for female sexual development and function, such as breast growth and the menstrual cycle. It helps regulate body temperature and blood pressure, improve mood, enhance energy, and increase sexual interest. Listed below are other overall functions of estrogen:

- Aids in formation of the brain's neurotransmitters, which decrease depression, irritability, and anxiety (see Chapter 18 for more about neurotransmitters and weight gain)

- Decreases arterial plaque

- Decreases LDLs ("bad" cholesterol)

- Decreases wrinkles

- Helps maintain memory

- Helps prevent tooth loss

- Helps with fine motor skills

- Improves insulin sensitivity

- Increases blood flow

- Increases concentration

- Increases HDLs ("good" cholesterol)

- Increases metabolic rate

- Maintains bone density

- Maintains collagen in skin

- Reduces overall risk of heart disease

- Reduces risk of cataracts

There are three types of estrogen that a woman produces naturally—estrone, estradiol, and estriol. It is important to know a little about these estrogens in order to understand their role in affecting weight, which is discussed later in this chapter.

Before menopause, *estrone* (E1) is made primarily by the ovaries, where it is converted to estradiol (the strongest estrogen). After menopause, because the function of the ovaries greatly decreases, estrone is made primarily in the fat cells and is converted into estradiol at a greatly reduced rate.

Estradiol (E2) is the most potent and predominant estrogen that women produce before menopause. It plays a crucial role in the menstrual cycle and is responsible for the development of secondary sexual characteristics, such as breast development and the growth of underarm and pubic hair. These changes begin at the time of puberty and are enhanced during the reproductive years. As already explained, estradiol production is greatly reduced after menopause.

Estriol (E3) is considered the weakest of the estrogens compared to estrone and estradiol. It is produced in significant amounts only during pregnancy.

When estrogen is not in correct balance with other hormones (primarily progesterone), weight gain is a common result. Extra pounds, especially around the abdomen, hips, and thighs, are common signs of excess estrogen. Other common symptoms that can also have a direct effect on weight gain include water retention, abdominal bloating, fatigue, and depression.

Progesterone

Progesterone, which is necessary for balancing estrogen levels, plays an important role in menstruation, pregnancy, and the formation of embryos. It has a direct effect on weight, as it helps the body use and eliminate fat, enhances the action of thyroid hormones, and increases metabolism. In addition to the functions just listed, progesterone has a number of other roles, including the following:

- Balances fluid in the cells

- Has a natural calming effect

- Has a positive effect on sleep patterns

- Helps build bone

- Increases scalp hair

- Inhibits breast tissue overgrowth (may protect against breast cancer)

- Is a natural antidepressant

- Lowers cholesterol

- Lowers high blood pressure

- Relaxes the smooth muscle in the gut so the body can break down food into nutrients

When the body produces too much progesterone, fat storage increases, as does appetite—for carbohydrates in particular. Elevated progesterone is also linked to high cortisol levels and increased insulin production (and insulin resistance)—both of which are connected to weight gain. (For more on how cortisol and insulin resistance affect weight, see Chapters 6 and 16, respectively.)

Testosterone

Testosterone falls into a class of hormones called *androgens*. Androgens are commonly referred to as "male" hormones because the human characteristics they stimulate and control—such as muscles, hair growth, and deepening of the voice—are considered masculine. Although testosterone is the principal male sex hormone, it is also present to a lesser degree in females, who produce about half of it in the ovaries and half in the adrenal glands. Its functions include the following:

- Elevates norepinephrine in the brain (has same effect as taking an antidepressant)

- Helps decrease excess body fat

- Helps increase metabolism

- Helps increase muscle mass and tone

- Helps maintain bone strength

- Helps maintain memory

- Increases sense of self-confidence and emotional well-being

- Increases sexual interest

Weight gain is a common result when testosterone is not produced in proper amounts. Reduced levels are less effective in helping limit the storage of body fat, while its role in increasing metabolism is also compromised. High levels commonly lead to insulin resistance, which is discussed in Chapter 16.

WHICH FEMALE HORMONAL CONDITIONS CONTRIBUTE TO WEIGHT GAIN?

A number of female conditions that are affected by hormone imbalance are associated with weight gain, including premenstrual syndrome (PMS), polycystic ovarian syndrome (PCOS), and perimenopause/menopause. What follows are overviews of these conditions, including what they are, how they contribute to weight gain, and what you can do to avoid putting on those unwanted pounds.

PREMENSTRUAL SYNDROME (PMS)

Affecting between 60 to 75 percent of women in the United States, premenstrual syndrome (PMS) is characterized by the recurrence of physical and/or psychological symptoms during the days (or weeks) prior to the menstrual cycle. This means that as many as three out of every four women who menstruate experience some form of PMS.

Although the exact cause or causes of PMS are not known, changes in hormone levels during the menstrual cycle are considered important factors. Low progesterone levels on days twelve through fourteen of the cycle (confirmed by a saliva test) are commonly associated with PMS, and often result in irritability, anxiety, and depression. Estrogen levels decrease both at ovulation and just before the cycle begins. A decrease in estrogen levels affects your neurotransmitters—serotonin and dopamine levels decline, which can lead to depression, while norepinephrine levels may increase, making you feel more anxious and irritable.

There are other factors that are believed to contribute to PMS, such as low blood sugar levels and caffeine consumption. Taking oral contraceptives, which contain progestin (synthetic progesterone), is another. Nutrition can also play a role. Deficiencies in certain vitamins and minerals, such as vitamin B_6, calcium, and magnesium, can make PMS symptoms worse. Eating salty foods can cause water retention, while drinking alcohol can cause mood and energy disturbances, which can also aggravate symptoms.

What Are the Symptoms of PMS?

Dozens of signs and symptoms are associated with PMS. Some of these symptoms, such as intestinal bloating, appetite changes, and salt and sugar cravings, have a direct effect on weight gain. The following list, although not complete, includes other common symptoms:

- Aches and pains
- Anxiety
- Backache
- Breast tenderness
- Cramps
- Depression
- Diarrhea/constipation

- Difficulty concentrating
- Fatigue
- Food sensitivity
- Headaches
- Insomnia
- Irritability
- Mood swings

While the reported number of symptoms is overwhelming, in actuality, most women who have PMS experience only a few. And for most, the problems occur in predictable patterns, although the symptoms may be more severe during some months.

How Do You Determine if You Have PMS?

Because it is associated with so many signs and symptoms, which typically subside once the cycle begins, PMS can be difficult to diagnose. The only factor the symptoms have in common is that they occur on the days before the monthly period. There is no test to positively diagnose PMS. Doctors may attribute symptoms to PMS based upon your premenstrual pattern.

How Does PMS Contribute to Weight Gain?

Every woman's body is different. Although some women with PMS may not experience weight gain at all, for many others, it is a common complaint. Most women gain between two and five pounds during this time. The good news is that this weight is generally gone within a few days. But what are some of the reasons for it?

For starters, fluctuating estrogen and progesterone levels have a direct effect on appetite. PMS is a time of cravings, especially for sweet and salty foods. Is anything more satisfying than giving into these desires with a luscious bar of chocolate or a bowl of salty potato chips? Not only does giving into these cravings add calories, it may also curb your appetite for healthier food choices. Furthermore, an increased salt intake will cause your body to retain water.

Feeling stressed and irritable during PMS is another common result of hormonal imbalance. As levels of estrogen rise and fall, stress levels (cortisol) increase, which stimulates the appetite, especially for carbohydrates and fatty foods. Furthermore, anxiety and irritability often go hand in hand during times of stress, and eating is one of the ways in which you may soothe yourself into feeling better.

While experiencing PMS, many women who exercise regularly, stop their usual routine because they feel crampy and bloated and would rather stay on the couch. If you find yourself in this situation, be aware that avoiding your usual exercise regimen may cause that added PMS weight to stick around—especially if you've also been giving in to your cravings for calorie-laden snacks.

What Can You Do to Reduce or Avoid PMS Weight Gain?

Keeping off the PMS pounds may be a lot easier than you think. There are a few steps you can take to reduce or, in some instances, even avoid weight gain during this time.

From a dietary standpoint, making a few changes in your eating habits can help limit those extra pounds. Eating smaller meals more frequently and limiting your intake of salty foods can reduce water retention and bloating. Eating fruits, vegetables, whole grains, and calcium-rich foods are recommended. Pineapple, bananas, and other potassium-rich foods help reduce intestinal bloating. Increasing your intake of high-fiber foods, which keep you feeling full, will help curb your appetite. When your appetite is in check, you won't be as likely to give into cravings, but if you must indulge, try not to overdo it. Also consider healthier choices. Instead of eating that bar (or two) of chocolate, opt for a few chocolate-covered strawberries or a scoop of chocolate frozen yogurt.

Avoiding caffeine and alcohol also helps, as does drinking lots of water. Not only does water help keep you hydrated and fill you up, it actually helps eliminate those unwanted pounds. (To learn more about this, see Chapter 7.) Exercising regularly is another way to reduce and help manage PMS symptoms. Incorporating thirty minutes of daily exercise several times a week can improve symptoms like fatigue and depressed mood, which for many women, are associated with an increased appetite and food cravings.

As discussed in Chapter 6, stress can be a major contributor to weight gain, not only when experiencing premenstrual syndrome, but at any time. Try to relax more and spend time doing the things that you truly enjoy. Making sure you get enough sleep is one way to lower stress; muscle relaxation exercises, deep breathing techniques, yoga, and massages are others. Taking nice long walks will also work off some of the tension you may be feeling.

Another way to treat PMS is by taking the appropriate nutritional supplements. The table found below provides a number of supplements that can be effective in treating a variety of PMS symptoms, including those that may contribute to weight gain.

SUPPLEMENTS TO TREAT PMS		
Supplement	Dosage	Considerations
B-complex vitamins	Choose a B-complex vitamin that provides 10 to 50 mg each of vitamins B_1, B_2, B_3, B_5, and B_6; 200 to 400 mcg of folic acid; and 250 to 500 mcg of B_{12}. Take twice a day.	Speak to your health-care provider before taking if you have diabetes, liver problems, or anemia. B-complex vitamins may interact with certain antibiotics and anti-seizure medications. Whenever taking a B-complex vitamin, always take a multivitamin as well.
Black cohosh	20 mg twice a day.	Do not take if you have breast cancer, are pregnant, or are breastfeeding. Do not use if you are taking an antidepressant. Use with caution if you have high blood pressure.
Borage oil	500 mg twice a day.	Can help reduce breast tenderness, fluid retention, cramps, and psychological PMS symptoms.
Calcium	• 500 mg once a day for premenopausal women. • 800 mg once a day for perimenopausal women. • 1,000 mg once a day for menopausal women.	Although most people are deficient in calcium, there is a danger in taking too much. Do not ingest more than 1,000 to 1,200 mg of calcium a day.
Chasteberry	20 mg two to three times a day.	Do not take if you have breast cancer, are pregnant, or are breastfeeding.
Evening primrose	1,000 mg once or twice a day.	May cause stomach upset.
Ginkgo (*Ginkgo biloba*)	120 mg once a day.	Do not take if you are on a blood-thinning medication.

Magnesium	400 to 800 mg once a day.*	Consult health-care provider for dosage if you have kidney disease. Discontinue use and see your doctor if you experience abdominal pain. Take a lower dose if it causes diarrhea. Magnesium's citrate, glycinate, gluconate, and lactate forms are more easily absorbed than its oxide form.
Multivitamin, pharmaceutical-grade†	Follow the directions on the bottle.	Make sure to take only a pharmaceutical-grade multivitamin.
Omega-3 essential fatty acids EPA/DHA (fish oil)	2,000 to 10,000 mg once a day.*	In dosages above 4,000 mg, may cause the blood to thin. Do not take more than 4,000 mg a day if you are using a blood-thinning medication.
St. John's Wort (*Hypericum perforatum*)	300 to 400 mg three times a day.*	Do not take with antidepressants, indinavir, cyclosporine, theophylline, warfarin, or ethinylestradiol. If you are exposed to the sun, it may cause a skin rash. May lessen the effects of birth control pills.
Taurine	500 to 1,000 mg once a day.*	Take between meals. Do not take with aspirin or any salicylate. Check with your health-care provider before taking taurine if you have kidney disease. Discontinue use if you suddenly have feelings of chest or throat tightness or if you break out in hives.
Vitamin A and mixed carotenoids	5,000 IU—half vitamin A and half mixed carotenoids—once a day.	Use caution when taking vitamin A supplements because they have the potential to be toxic. Do not take high doses if you have liver disease, are a smoker, or have been exposed to asbestos.
Vitamin E	100 to 400 IU a day.*	Do not take with ferrous sulfate iron supplements, which destroy vitamin E. Do not take if you are on a blood-thinning medication. Take mixed tocopherols, the more active type of vitamin E.

*To choose an appropriate dose, see page 199 for information on dosage ranges.
† See page 197 for information on pharmaceutical-grade supplements.

Since PMS is affected by low progesterone levels, some women have found supplementation with progesterone to be helpful. It is important to supplement with bioidentical (natural) progesterone, which has the same chemical structure as the progesterone your body makes. The prescription, which is prepared by a compounding pharmacy, is to be used on days twelve through twenty-four of the menstrual cycle—days on which progesterone is characteristically low in women who experience PMS. For most women, this is applied transdermally (on the skin). If, however, you suffer from insomnia, it is best to take this progesterone in pill form, which has a calming effect that will allow you to sleep better. If you are considering supplementation, be sure to have your hormone levels tested by a qualified physician, preferably one who specializes in metabolic and anti-aging medicine. (See page 211 of the "Resources" section for organizations that can guide you to physicians in your area.) If you begin taking progesterone and you do not need it, you can very easily gain weight.

Some women have normal levels of progesterone, but low levels of estradiol (E2)—the strongest form of estrogen (see page 127). Low levels of E2 can affect serotonin production, which may trigger depression and changes in eating patterns. For these women, progesterone supplementation will not work, but the nutritional supplements recommended in the table above may be more effective.

As you can see, there are many options for reducing the discomfort of PMS and alleviating its symptoms, many of which can cause unwanted weight gain. Of course, before trying any of these remedies, *always* check with your health-care provider.

POLYCYSTIC OVARIAN SYNDROME (PCOS)

Polycystic ovarian syndrome (PCOS), a leading cause of infertility, occurs when the ovaries do not produce hormones in the proper balance for the eggs to fully mature. Instead of releasing a mature egg during ovulation, some of the follicles remain in the ovaries and become tiny fluid-filled cysts. PCOS, which affects as many as one in fifteen women, is characterized by irregular or absent menstrual cycles and excess testosterone (androgen) production. Many women with this condition are also overweight, and many are obese. If left untreated, PCOS can lead to serious health issues such as diabetes and heart disease.

Many scientists believe that PCOS has a hereditary component. There is also some suggestion that women with PCOS are born with a gene that triggers elevated levels of testosterone or insulin. Stress is believed to be another contributing factor to the development of PCOS. Recent studies have shown that many women with this condition cannot effectively process the stress hormone cortisol. This may lead to elevated cortisol levels and result in more stress. As seen in Chapter 6, prolonged levels of excess cortisol are associated with a number of symptoms that are connected to weight gain.

What Are the Symptoms of PCOS?

Signs and symptoms of PCOS usually begin during the teen years, vary from woman to woman, and can include:

- Acne
- Craving for carbohydrates
- Depression
- Elevated insulin levels
- High blood pressure
- Hirsutism (excessive facial/body hair)
- Infertility/recurrent miscarriages
- Irregular or absent menstrual cycles
- Obesity
- Oily skin
- Ovarian cysts

Any of these signs and symptoms may be absent in PCOS, with the exception of irregular or lack of menstrual periods. Women with PCOS commonly do not ovulate regularly.

How Do You Determine if You Have PCOS?

There is no single test to diagnose PCOS. If you are experiencing any of the associated symptoms, it is important to see a doctor to get a proper diagnosis. The doctor will ask questions about your general health, symptoms, and menstrual cycles. He or she will complete a physical exam to check for signs of PCOS, such as high blood pressure or excess body hair. The doctor will also check your body mass index (BMI) to determine if you are at an appropriate weight. Finally, various lab tests will be performed to assess levels of blood sugar, insulin, and other hormones. This will help rule out other hormonal problems that may have similar symptoms. A salivary test for hormonal levels may also be helpful.

Your doctor should be able to diagnose PCOS without performing a pelvic ultrasound. However, this test may be conducted to see if ovarian cysts are present.

How Does PCOS Contribute to Weight Gain?

For women with PCOS, excessive weight is a common symptom. Studies have shown that women with this condition store more fat and burn calories at a slower rate than other women. One of the most important underlying factors in PCOS is insulin resistance.

As explained in Chapter 16, insulin resistance is a condition that prevents the cells from absorbing glucose properly. Instead, the glucose remains in the bloodstream and is converted into fat, which is then stored in the body, usually in the abdomen and buttocks. This condition may also impair the body's ability to convert the amino acid tryptophan into the brain chemical serotonin, which is helpful in reducing food cravings.

Another reason weight gain is common in many women with PCOS is that, as mentioned earlier, they have trouble effectively processing cortisol, which is responsible for balancing blood sugar. Increased cortisol production hinders this ability.

What Can You Do to Lose Weight?

There is no cure for PCOS, but there are steps you can take to help manage it. A variety of treatment methods for this disorder can be effective in helping lower high insulin levels (which have a direct effect on weight loss), regulating the menstrual cycle, and reducing your chances of getting heart disease and diabetes. Many women may need a combination of treatments to meet these goals.

Because of the role that high insulin levels and insulin resistance play in PCOS, most women respond well to modifications in their diet and exercise program. The standard low-fat high-carbohydrate weight loss diet may not be the best approach for women with PCOS. High intakes of carbohydrates, especially refined carbohydrates (such as processed breads, crackers, white rice), will turn to sugar quickly, causing elevated insulin levels. Instead, try to eat a heart-healthy diet that is rich in fiber and contains foods that are low on the glycemic index (GI). Foods with a low GI ranking break down slowly during digestion. In turn, they release glucose slowly into the bloodstream, which helps keep insulin levels balanced. Eating lots of fresh vegetables and fruits, beans, nuts, and whole grains is recommended. Lentils, chickpeas, and broccoli specifically are very helpful in decreasing insulin levels. (For more on the glycemic index, see page 156 of Chapter 16.)

Regular exercise can help lower some of the risk factors associated with PCOS. Because exercise is effective in reducing insulin levels, it can be helpful in losing weight—and just about any type of exercise is beneficial. So try to find an activity or sport that you enjoy. (See Chapter 2 for more about exercise.) Since exercise can be especially helpful in lowering insulin levels after a meal, at the very least, consider taking a walk after lunch or dinner.

In an effort to control the weight gain associated with PCOS, your doctor may prescribe diabetes medications to help regulate insulin and blood sugar levels. The nutritional supplements listed in the table below can also be useful in managing these symptoms.

SUPPLEMENTS TO TREAT PCOS		
Supplement	Dosage	Considerations
Alpha-lipoic acid	100 mg once a day.	Improves blood sugar levels, so diabetics may be able to take less medication. If you have diabetes and are taking alpha-lipoic acid, check your blood sugar regularly.
B-complex vitamins	Choose a B-complex vitamin that provides 10 to 50 mg each of vitamins B_1, B_2, B_3, B_5, and B_6; 200 to 400 mcg of folic acid; and 250 to 500 mcg of B_{12}. Take twice a day.	Speak to your health-care provider before taking if you have diabetes, liver problems, or anemia. B-complex vitamins may interact with certain antibiotics and anti-seizure medications. Whenever taking a B-complex vitamin, always take a multivitamin as well.
Biotin	1 to 3 mg once a day.*	Use with caution if you have a duodenal or peptic ulcer and recurrent gastritis.
Chromium	400 mcg once a day.	Combining chromium with the protein picolinate allows your body to absorb the nutrient more efficiently. If you have kidney disease, consult your physician before taking chromium.
Cinnamon bark extract	100 mg once a day.	Cinnamon can lower your blood sugar. If you are taking a medication for blood sugar control, check your blood sugar levels and make adjustments as necessary. A lower dosage of medication may be needed.
CLA (conjugated linoleic acid)	1,000 mg three times a day.	Do not take for more than three months.

Coenzyme Q$_{10}$	60 to 200 mg once a day. If you are using over 100 mg a day, take in divided doses.*	May reduce the effects of blood-thinning medication. May cause diarrhea in dosages above 100 mg once a day.
Copper	1 to 3 mg once a day.*	Your copper-to-zinc ratio is important for your health. Always take zinc if you are taking copper. Do not take copper if you have Wilson's disease. Do not take the cupric oxide form, which has low bioavailability.
Fenugreek	500 mg three times a day.	Can cause bloating, diarrhea, and/or indigestion. May cause urine to smell sweet. Do not take if you are on a blood-thinning medication.
Gymnema sylvestre	200 mg twice a day.	Can reduce blood sugar levels, so exercise caution if you are taking a medication that lowers blood sugar.
Magnesium	400 to 800 mg once a day.*	Consult health-care provider for dosage if you have kidney disease. Discontinue use and see your doctor if you experience abdominal pain. Take a lower dose if it causes diarrhea. The citrate, glycinate, gluconate, and lactate forms are more easily absorbed than the oxide form.
Manganese	2 to 5 mg once a day.*	If you have chronic liver disease, consult with a physician before taking.
Multivitamin, pharmaceutical-grade†	Follow the directions on the bottle.	Make sure to take only a pharmaceutical-grade multivitamin.
Taurine	500 to 1,000 mg once a day.*	Take between meals. Do not take with aspirin or any salicylate. Check with your health-care provider before taking taurine if you have kidney disease. Discontinue use if you suddenly have feelings of chest or throat tightness or if you break out in hives.
Vanadium	20 to 50 mg once a day.*	Do not take more than 50 mg a day.
Vitamin C	1,000 mg once a day.	Doses higher than 5,000 mg may cause diarrhea. Mineral ascorbates and Ester-C are buffered forms that lower the chance of diarrhea. Don't take high doses if you are prone to kidney stones or gout.
Vitamin D	To determine proper dosage, have your doctor measure your vitamin D levels. The minimum dose prescribed should be 400 IU.	In excessive amounts, vitamin D can be toxic. Do not exceed the dose prescribed by your physician.

| Zinc | 25 mg once a day. | The best-absorbed zinc supplements are zinc picolinate and zinc citrate. Side effects of zinc supplements may include nausea, stomach upset, and heartburn. If these effects persist or worsen, notify your doctor promptly. |

*To choose an appropriate dose, see page 199 for information on dosage ranges.
†See page 197 for information on pharmaceutical-grade supplements.

Also be aware that high doses of niacin, a B vitamin that occurs naturally in plants and animals and is available as a supplement, should be avoided by people with PCOS as it can worsen insulin sensitivity.

It is important to keep in mind that if you suffer from PCOS, losing weight in itself can be helpful in treating this disorder. Dropping as little as 5 percent of your total weight can be effective in leveling out hormonal imbalances and normalizing insulin levels.

PERIMENOPAUSE/MENOPAUSE

Every day in the United States, 3,500 women enter menopause, which is defined as the permanent end of menstruation and fertility. Menopause occurs naturally in women when the ovaries begin making less estrogen and progesterone, which were previously involved in regulating the menstrual cycle. Women can begin to experience menopause symptoms as early as fifteen years prior to actual menopause.

Perimenopause is the time when your body begins its transition into menopause. It usually starts anywhere from two to eight years before menopause and lasts up until the first year after your final menstrual period. Your estrogen and progesterone levels rise and fall unevenly during this time. You may still have menstrual cycles, but they might become more irregular. Also, the amount of menstrual blood during each cycle may be lighter or heavier than what you've previously experienced. Menopause most commonly occurs between the ages of thirty-five and fifty-five.

What Are the Symptoms of Menopause?

Fluctuating hormones cause menopausal symptoms that vary in type and intensity from woman to woman. For many women, a menstrual cycle that becomes irregular and then stops is their only symptom. Others, however, experience more uncomfortable or unpleasant symptoms like hot flashes, night sweats, and mood swings. For most women, menopause is a time of weight gain. The following list includes other common symptoms:

- Abdominal bloating
- Aching ankles, knees, wrists, shoulders, and heels
- Decreased sexual interest
- Depression
- Facial hair growth
- Flatulence (gas)
- Frequent urination
- Hair loss
- Hot flashes
- Indigestion
- Insomnia
- Irritability
- Loss of focus and concentration
- Lower back pain

- Memory lapses
- Migraine headaches
- Mood swings
- Night sweats
- Osteoporosis or osteopenia
- Painful intercourse
- Palpitations
- Panic attacks
- Snoring
- Sore breasts
- Urinary leakage
- Urinary tract infections
- Vaginal dryness
- Vaginal itching
- Vaginal odor
- Varicose veins

Although this list of symptoms may seem overwhelming, fortunately, most women will experience only a few. For some, these symptoms can last from a few months to many years.

How Do You Determine if You Are Experiencing Menopause?

The diagnosis of menopause is based upon your lack of a menstrual cycle for twelve consecutive months. Through blood tests, your doctor may also check your levels of luteinizing hormone (LH) and follicle stimulating hormone (FSH). Production of these hormones, which help regulate the menstrual cycle and egg production, increases as menopause occurs.

How Does Menopause Contribute to Weight Gain?

As your body winds down from its reproductive phase and heads toward menopause, estrogen production really starts to decline. As your ovaries produce less estrogen, your body looks to get it from other sources—and your fat cells are the primary source. Earlier in this chapter, you learned that the body naturally produces three types of estrogen. During the reproductive years, estrone (E1) is made primarily by the ovaries, where it is converted to estradiol (the strongest estrogen). After menopause, however, because the function of the ovaries greatly decreases, estrone is made primarily in the fat cells. Since fat cells can generate estrogen, your body works harder to convert calories into fat. Unfortunately, the more fat you have, the slower your metabolism becomes. And unlike muscle cells, fat cells don't burn calories efficiently. The body ends up storing more fat than it used to, and those unwanted pounds start to accumulate. Most of this weight comes on gradually during perimenopause and typically settles around your abdomen.

Progesterone levels also decrease during menopause. Lower levels can be responsible for water retention and bloating. And testosterone, which helps your body burn calories and create lean muscle mass, also may decline during this time. When these levels drop, your body produces less muscle, experiences a slowdown in metabolism, and more easily stores food as fat. And if cortisol levels increase at this time (typically due to stress), you will store more fat, lose muscle mass, and increase the chances of insulin resistance.

What Can You Do to Lose Weight?

To regain hormonal balance and combat menopausal weight gain, hormone replacement therapy (HRT) can be successful. HRT replenishes the body with the hormones in which it is deficient. The goal is not only to alleviate symptoms of menopause, but also to prevent serious health conditions like osteoporosis and heart disease. Research has shown that women who take HRT and are hormonally balanced tend to gain less weight than women who don't. (For more information on HRT, see the inset "Before Beginning Hormone Replacement" on page 142.)

Although a certain amount of weight gain during menopause is normal, it is important to avoid gaining excess amounts. One of the best strategies is to increase your body's metabolism, which tends to become sluggish primarily due to fluctuating levels of estrogen, progesterone, and testosterone. Maintaining a regular exercise program that incorporates weight training and aerobic exercises is an effective way to improve your body's metabolism.

Before Beginning Hormone Replacement

If you are interested in beginning hormone replacement therapy (HRT) to treat hormonal imbalance, be aware that the therapy you need will be as individualized as your own fingerprints. When it comes to HRT, "one size fits all" does *not* apply.

Begin by choosing a qualified health-care practitioner. My strong recommendation is that you work with a physician who specializes in metabolic and anti-aging medicine. In order to assess your individual hormonal needs, he or she will measure all of your hormone levels, usually through saliva or urine testing. Based on test results, your practitioner will prescribe a hormone supplement—often a combination of hormones—to meet your specific needs.

Be aware that the best hormone substitutes are bioidentical (natural) hormones, not synthetic. Bioidentical hormones have the exact same chemical structure as the hormones your body produces. For individualized dosing, prescriptions are prepared by compounding pharmacies.

Once you have begun HRT, your hormone levels should be measured again, usually after three months. Subsequent tests should be performed on a routine basis depending on your own personal needs and your body's response to therapy.

Making good food choices is another key component to losing excess weight during this time. Eating frequent small meals throughout the day that include foods with low rankings on the glycemic index (GI) will help keep your insulin levels balanced. Avoid starches, sugary foods, and refined products, which cause spikes in insulin levels, followed by drops that result in strong appetite cravings. (For more on the glycemic index, see Chapter 16.) Consume healthy fats containing omega-3s, such as nuts and monounsaturated oil, and choose whole grains and fiber-rich foods, which help keep you full and satisfied. (For more information on dietary fats, see the inset "A Primer on Good and Bad Fats" found on page 73 of Chapter 9.)

A number of nutritional supplements have been effective in treating some of the symptoms of perimenopause/menopause. They are listed in the table on page 143.

SUPPLEMENTS TO TREAT PERIMENOPAUSE/MENOPAUSE

Supplement	Dosage	Considerations
Black cohosh	20 mg twice a day.	Do not take if you have breast cancer, are pregnant, or are breastfeeding. Do not use if you are taking an antidepressant. Use with caution if you have high blood pressure.
Chasteberry	20 mg two to three times a day.	Do not take if you have breast cancer, are pregnant, or are breastfeeding.
Dong quai	3 to 10 grams once a day.*	Do not take if you have breast cancer, are pregnant, or are breastfeeding. Do not take if you have the cold or flu, or if you have diarrhea. Do not use if you are taking blood thinners. May cause a rash if you are exposed to the sun. Also may interfere with the following herbs: garlic, ginger, ginkgo, ginseng, licorice, skullcap, and turmeric.

*To choose an appropriate dose, see page 199 for information on dosage ranges.

It is important to keep in mind that menopause is a natural phase in life. A few extra pounds can actually be helpful in lessening the anxiety, hot flashes, and other uncomfortable symptoms that are commonly associated with menopause. What is most important during this time is a focus on eating right, exercising regularly, and maintaining a healthy lifestyle.

CONCLUSION

If an imbalance or deficiency in female hormones is preventing you from losing weight, there are many things you can do to improve your body's balance of these essential chemicals. Dietary modifications, exercise, stress-reduction techniques, nutritional supplementation, and possibly hormone replacement therapy can help reduce symptoms, improve your overall health, and enable you to reach your desired weight.

On the other hand, female hormonal dysfunction may be just one of several factors that are preventing you from shedding pounds. If you take steps to treat the conditions associated with hormonal problems and are still not able to lose those extra pounds, be sure to explore the other chapters in this book, each of which examines a specific lifestyle issue, health problem, or biochemical factor that may be affecting your efforts to reduce Once you have identified the contributing factors, turn to Chapter 20, "Putting It All Together," which will help you create an integrated weight-loss program that is suited to your needs.

15

Genes

Peaple come in different physical packages—short or tall, dark- or light-skinned, with eyes that range from the palest blue to the deepest brown. For over a century, scientists have known that these visible traits are determined by inherited genes. But only in the last few decades have researchers recognized that genes play a role not only in how the body looks, but also how it functions. And only in the last few years has it become apparent that genes have a very real effect on body weight and the weight-loss process. Specific genes can make it more likely that some people will put on extra weight, and even influence the way they lose (or don't lose) those added pounds.

Although you can't change the genes that were handed down to you by your parents, it is possible to lose weight despite your inherited traits. And in some cases, understanding the way genes work can actually help you shed pounds with greater ease and success. Before you learn how genes work, though, it's helpful to know a little bit about what they are.

WHAT ARE GENES?

To learn about genes, you have to look inside human cells, which are the building blocks of human life. The body is made up of trillions of cells, and each cell has a *nucleus*—a control center that regulates cell activity. All of the genetic contents of the cell are found within this nucleus in the form of *DNA* (*deoxyribonucleic acid*), which is a huge chemical database that carries the instructions for making all the proteins the cells will ever need. In short, human DNA is a blueprint for building a human being.

DNA carries its genetic information in segments called *genes*. Each gene contains a particular set of instructions, or codes, that allow a cell to produce a specific protein, usually an enzyme, that starts one specific activity in the cell. By initiating and regulating these activities, it is the genes, controlled by the nucleus, that establish each individual's traits—appearance, growth and development, and (to an extent) behavior.

Each person has two copies of each gene, one inherited from each parent. A few traits, such as colorblindness, are determined by a single gene inherited from the mother or father. But most genetic traits, such as the shape of the nose, are determined by interactions between several genes. In these cases, both the mother's and father's genes may come into play. Because everyone has approximately 25,000 separate genes, a nearly endless number of combinations are possible.

Only a fraction of each cell's genes are *expressed*, or turned on. The remainder are *repressed*, or turned off. This process of gene regulation is what enables a kidney cell, for instance, to develop differently from a brain cell even though the two cells contain the same genes. It also allows cells to react quickly to alterations in their environment. Although experts know that the regulation of genes is necessary for life and is occurring all the time, they do not fully understand the complex process involved.

The story of genes is complicated by the fact that these coded bits of information are not always passed from generation to generation unaltered. Instead, *mutations*—physical changes in genetic material—sometimes take place. *Hereditary* or *germline mutations* are either passed down from parent to child or occur at the beginning of a human life, when eggs or sperm develop a change. Other mutations can be acquired during a person's lifetime in response to environmental pressures such as ultraviolet radiation or random errors in cell division. Mutated genes may be benign or malignant. A *benign mutation* is a harmless change that affects a trait such as eye color. A *malignant mutation* can cause a disorder such as cancer.

WHAT ARE THE SYMPTOMS OF GENETIC PROBLEMS?

There are no specific symptoms which indicate that your genes may be contributing to your weight problems. But if you find that you don't feel full and satisfied even after eating a big meal, that you put weight on despite dietary restrictions, or that proven weight-loss diets do not enable you to shed pounds, genetic factors may be at work. If you have a parent or grandparent who has experienced similar weight problems, there is an even greater likelihood that genes have been contributing to your weight-loss difficulties.

HOW DO GENES CONTRIBUTE TO WEIGHT GAIN?

Beginning in the 1980s, researchers began to pinpoint specific genes as culprits in various disorders. This research was made easier by the government-sponsored Human Genome Project, which in 1990, began the work of mapping human DNA. (See the inset "The Human Genome Project" on page 148 for more information.) Scientists have now identified several genes that predispose individuals to gain weight or to lose weight only under certain circumstances.

One gene found to contribute to weight gain and obesity is the *FTO gene*. Researchers discovered that people who have two copies of this gene—a copy from each parent—are more than six pounds heavier on average than people who do not have the gene or who have only one copy, and are 67 percent more likely to become obese. This gene seems to be most common among people of European descent, but has also been found in people of Chinese descent and may be present in other ethnic groups as well. At this point, it is not certain whether the FTO gene promotes weight gain by causing people to eat more food, causing them to choose higher-calorie foods, or causing their bodies to store more fat.

Another gene that can play a part in obesity is the so-called *leptin gene*. Chapter 1 explained that leptin is a hormone secreted by the body to let your brain know that you have had enough to eat. Leptin, in other words, puts the brakes on eating, avoiding the excessive consumption of calories that can lead to weight gain and obesity. In some people, a mutation of the leptin gene keeps the body from producing or responding to this important hormone, leading to constant cravings for food. This, in turn, results in severe obesity. Fortunately, this genetic problem is extremely rare.

Genes can also play a part in obesity by affecting the way you perceive sweet and bitter tastes. Researchers now believe that taste does not end at the back of the tongue, as previously thought, but continues throughout the digestive tract and other tissues, where it helps regulate both appetite and blood sugar levels. These receptors also appear to direct the secretion of metabolic hormones in the lower digestive tract. Studies have even shown a genetic predisposition for "fat taste," which helps the body select foods that contain fat-soluble vitamins and essential fatty acids. In other words, genetic variations in taste may account for differences in your food choices and even help determine how much you eat.

Perhaps the most encouraging genetic discovery concerns genes that predispose people to respond better to either a low-carbohydrate diet or a low-fat diet. In studies involving overweight women, it was found that individuals with a genetic tendency to benefit from a low-carb diet lose two and a half times as much weight as people who follow the same diet but do not have this predisposition. Similarly, women predisposed to respond to a low-fat diet lose much more weight from that eating plan than women who follow the same diet but lack the low-fat gene. Among Caucasian women, studies indicate that 39 percent would benefit from a low-fat diet, while 45 percent should follow a low-carb diet.

Research into the connection between body weight and genes is still in its infancy, but progress continues to be made. Experts believe that there may be *hundreds* of genes related to weight gain and obesity. Future research in the subject will likely result in drugs that, by targeting the

The Human Genome Project

Formally begun in 1990 and completed in 2003—two years ahead of schedule—the Human Genome Project (HGP) was an international effort coordinated by the US Department of Energy and the National Institutes of Health. The project, which involved dozens of laboratories around the world, was designed to achieve a number of important goals, including:

- Identifying the thousands of genes—the *genome*—that make up human DNA

- Determining the sequences of the 3 billion chemical pairs that make up human DNA

- Storing this new information in a database

- Improving the tools used to analyze this data

- Addressing the ethical, legal, and social issues that may arise from gene research

The detailed knowledge that HGP produced on specific genes has already served as a springboard to research into the causes of numerous physical disorders, including obesity. As research continues, experts hope to improve our understanding of genetic conditions, create medications that effectively target the most fundamental causes of disease, and pinpoint ways to avoid the environmental factors that can trigger disease.

actions of specific genes, can help prevent excess weight or enable some dieters to lose pounds with greater ease.

HOW DO YOU DETERMINE IF GENES ARE AFFECTING YOUR WEIGHT?

Genetic testing is readily available through companies that specialize in this procedure. For instance, Pathway Genomics (see page 208 of "Resources") will send you a saliva collection kit that makes it easy to submit a sample for analysis. This, as well as a health survey that you fill out, will form the basis of the company's report, which will be available for your review in a matter of weeks. Your health-care provider will then be able to interpret your genetic profile so that you can better understand if your genes are having an impact on your ability to lose weight.

WHAT CAN YOU DO TO LOSE WEIGHT?

If you find that you are genetically predisposed to benefit from either a low-fat or low-carbohydrate diet, you are fortunate in that you can tailor your eating plan to suit your makeup. Just remember that you will increase the likelihood of losing weight if you include exercise as part of your strategy. (To learn more about exercise and weight loss, see Chapter 2.)

Even if you find that that your genetic makeup, or *genotype*, includes a trait that predisposes you to weight gain, you do not have to resign yourself to being overweight. In most cases, genes indicate a *tendency* but do not rule your destiny. Proof of this was found by researchers who studied 700 Amish people. It was discovered that many Amish men and women have two copies of the FTO gene, and therefore have an inherited tendency to gain excess weight, but that their high level of physical activity keeps them trim. The Amish lifestyle, which involves working hard every day on a farm, as well as other forms of physical labor, appears to override the FTO gene. Experts also believe that the Amish diet, which is rich in organic farm-raised vegetables and fruits, plays an important part in weight control.

Fortunately, you don't have to follow a traditional lifestyle to keep weight off or lose pounds. By boosting physical activity, choosing unprocessed foods, and making a conscious effort to limit portion sizes, you can achieve a healthy weight regardless of your genetic inheritance.

CONCLUSION

Genes are just one of the many factors that affect body weight, so even if these inherited traits are not on your side, you should not be discouraged. Studies have shown that that in most cases, your way of life is just as powerful as your DNA.

If your weight-loss efforts are not as successful as you'd like, be sure to explore the other chapters in this book, each of which examines a specific lifestyle issue, health problem, or biochemical factor that may be causing problems. Once you have identified the contributing factors, turn to Chapter 20, "Putting It All Together," which will help you create an integrated weight-loss program that is suited to your needs.

16

Insulin Resistance

The human body is a highly complex machine that, in order to exist, has to accomplish a range of important functions, including breathing, reproduction, circulation, and more. Every step of each one of these functions is regulated by chemical substances known as *hormones*. The body's messengers, hormones send signals to the cells so that they know what to do and when to do it. When the body makes the right amounts of hormones and these important chemicals do their job, you are healthy. When something goes wrong along the way—a hormone is not produced or the body doesn't respond to the message it sends—health problems can appear.

One of the most important functions of the body is the production of energy. This process, which takes places in the cells, fuels every other physiological activity needed to maintain life. The most important hormone in the control of energy production is the substance known as *insulin*. Usually, this chemical messenger works as it should and the body produces the energy it needs to survive. But sometimes, the body stops listening to its own messenger's signal and a disorder known as *insulin resistance* develops. When this occurs, a common result is excess weight.

Insulin resistance is not an unusual condition. Experts estimate that about 25 percent of all Americans, or 80 million people, suffer from insulin resistance, and the results can be devastating. In addition to weight gain, this disorder is associated with high blood pressure, high triglycerides, low HDL (the "good" cholesterol), and an increased risk of cancer. When left uncontrolled, insulin resistance is a risk factor for heart disease and type 2 diabetes. That's the bad news. The good news is that there are steps you can take to avoid and effectively treat this condition. The first step, of course, is understanding it.

WHAT IS INSULIN RESISTANCE?

In order to understand insulin resistance, you have to know a little about the key role that insulin performs in the body. When you eat, your digestive system breaks food down into *glucose*, a type of sugar that is the body's chief form of energy. The glucose is then transported through the bloodstream to cells throughout the body. As glucose levels rise, a signal is sent to the pancreas to create more insulin, causing blood insulin levels to rise as well. In a healthy body, the insulin then allows the sugar to move out of the bloodstream and into the cells, where it can be used. This is, in fact, insulin's most important role: It enables the body to process glucose into energy, which, in turn, fuels all the body's functions. But in the case of insulin resistance, the cells don't respond to the insulin messenger, and the glucose is prevented from entering the cells. The pancreas reacts by producing even *more* insulin, but since the cells have essentially closed their doors to the glucose, the additional insulin doesn't do any good. Many people with insulin resistance have elevated levels of both insulin and glucose. Every time they eat, the body produces more glucose; every time their glucose levels rise, the body secretes more insulin.

Some experts believe that insulin resistance develops in response to a diet that is high in carbohydrates, especially simple carbohydrates such as those found in white bread, candy, cakes, cookies, and other highly refined foods. When you eat simple carbs, sugars quickly enter the bloodstream, causing blood glucose levels to rise abruptly. The body then releases high levels of insulin to keep blood glucose levels under control. In some people, if insulin spikes too frequently, over time, the overworked cells become less responsive to the hormone, creating the condition known as insulin resistance. High levels of insulin, referred to as *hyperinsulimia*, can also be caused by the following factors:

- Abuse of alcohol
- Birth control pills or other progestins
- Decreased estrogen in women
- Decreased testosterone in men
- Elevated DHEA
- Excessive caffeine intake
- Excessive dieting
- Excessive progesterone in women
- Increased stress
- Increased testosterone in women

- Insomnia
- Hypothyroidism (underactive thyroid)
- Lack of exercise
- Nicotine

What Other Roles Does Insulin Play in the Body?

Insulin's most well-known role is to help cells absorb glucose and turn it into energy. But this is not the only function of insulin. This important hormone also:

- Decreases the production of disease-causing free radicals
- Dilates blood vessels
- Lowers blood pressure
- Reduces the incidence of atherosclerosis (the buildup of plaques on artery walls)
- Reduces inflammation
- Reduces the occurrence of blood clots

WHAT ARE THE SYMPTOMS OF INSULIN RESISTANCE?

When insulin resistance is mild, you may have no symptoms at all. If your condition is more severe, however, you may experience one or more of the following signs:

- Acne
- Ankle swelling
- Burning feet
- Confusion (brain fog)
- Constipation
- Dark, thickened areas of the skin, especially on the back of the neck
- Decreased memory
- Depression
- Fatigue
- Fluctuating high blood pressure
- Inability to focus
- Increased levels of triglycerides

- Infertility
- Intestinal bloating
- Irregular menstrual cycles
- Irritability
- Loose bowel movements alternating with constipation

- Sleepiness after meals
- Water retention
- Weight gain and fat storage, especially in the buttocks or abdomen

If several of these symptoms sound familiar to you, perhaps insulin resistance is contributing to your weight-loss problem.

HOW DOES INSULIN RESISTANCE CONTRIBUTE TO WEIGHT GAIN?

You now know that insulin resistance prevents cells from absorbing the glucose that enters the bloodstream as the result of digestion. When the cells fail to absorb the glucose, the levels of glucose in the blood remain abnormally high. Because the body is designed to keep glucose levels in a narrow range, it takes action to get the glucose under control in a different way: It signals the liver to convert the blood sugar into fat. This fat is then stored in the body, especially in the belly and buttocks.

Although the process through which insulin resistance leads to excess weight seems simple, it leads to a vicious cycle that is a little more complex. The body's cells, now starved for the glucose that they can't absorb, fail to produce energy, leading to feelings of exhaustion. In response, the body signals the individual to eat more, and especially causes it to crave the carbohydrate-rich foods that used to produce nearly instant energy. The carbohydrates lead to the production of more glucose, more insulin, and more fat cells. As the ratio of fat to muscle increases in the body, the body becomes less able to burn fat, making it more difficult to lose the recently acquired weight. Insulin resistance also impairs the body's ability to convert the amino acid tryptophan into the brain chemical serotonin. Because one of the functions of serotonin is to curb food cravings and shut off appetite, lower levels of the chemical increase the urge to eat, leading to yet more weight gain.

HOW DO YOU DETERMINE IF YOU ARE INSULIN RESISTANT?

There is no single test used to detect insulin resistance. But if clinical tests reveal high blood glucose levels, high levels of triglycerides and LDL ("bad") cholesterol, and decreased concentrations of HDL ("good") cholesterol, your doctor will suspect that your body has become unable to properly produce or utilize insulin. Standard blood tests show levels of triglycerides, LDL cholesterol, and HDL cholesterol. To determine blood glucose levels, your doctor may order one of the following procedures.

- **Glycated Hemoglobin (A1C) Test.** By measuring the percentage of blood sugar attached to your hemoglobin after fasting, this blood test shows your average blood glucose level for the past several months. An A1C level between 5.7 and 6.5 percent indicates that you may have *pre-diabetes* (a condition that may lead to diabetes), and that you may be insulin resistant.

- **Fasting Blood Sugar Test.** For this test, a blood sample is taken after you fast for at least eight hours or overnight. A fasting blood sugar level above 90 mg/dL (milligrams per deciliter) indicates that you are headed toward prediabetes. A fasting blood sugar level from 100 to 125 mg/dL indicates prediabetes.

- **Oral Glucose Tolerance Test.** For this test, a blood sample is taken after you fast for eight hours or overnight, and then drink a sugary solution. Sometimes referred to as an *impaired glucose tolerance test (IGT)*, this procedure indicates prediabetes if the blood sugar level is 140 to 199 mg/dL.

If your doctor finds that you have high blood glucose levels, depending on the degree of the problem, lifestyle changes and/or medication may be advised. The dietary modifications that are recommended in the following section can help you in your efforts to control high blood sugar and insulin resistance, and, in the process, assist you in losing any unwanted pounds.

WHAT CAN YOU DO TO LOSE WEIGHT?

If you suspect that insulin resistance is contributing to your difficulty in losing weight, the best way to start treatment is to follow a nutritionally sound diet. Earlier in this chapter, you learned about the link between insulin resistance and carbohydrates. When your diet includes a lot of refined carbohydrates, your bloodstream is continually flooded with glu-

156 · Why You Can't Lose Weight

cose, making it difficult to control blood glucose levels. Yet the body requires carbohydrates to function. In fact, the best diet for most people is 40 percent carbohydrates, 35 percent protein, and 25 percent healthy fat. What's the answer? You need to choose *healthy* carbs—carbs that are low on the glycemic index.

Created to help diabetes patients manage their blood sugar level, the *glycemic index* (GI) ranks foods according to the effect that their particular carbohydrates have on blood glucose. Foods that have a low GI ranking contain a carbohydrate that breaks down slowly during digestion, causing a gradual release of glucose into the bloodstream. These are the foods that should make up the bulk of your carbohydrate consumption. You want to avoid foods that have a high GI value and will therefore break down more quickly, causing an undesirable surge of blood glucose and a resulting rise in insulin. Foods with moderate GI rankings should be eaten in moderation. The following table, which lists low, moderate, and high GI foods, can help you plan a diet that can control or even eliminate insulin resistance.

GLYCEMIC INDEX FOOD RATINGS
Low Glycemic Index Foods

All-Bran cereal	Cannellini beans	Navy beans
Apples	Cantaloupe	Oranges
Apricots, dried	Carob	Pasta, whole wheat
Baked beans	Celery	Peaches
Bananas	Cherries	Pears
Barley	Chickpeas	Peas
Bell peppers	Corn	Plums
Black beans	Grapefruit	Potato chips
Blackberries	Grapes	Raspberries
Black-eyed peas	Green beans	Rye
Blueberries	Green peas	Soybeans
Bread, whole grain	Kidney beans	Spaghetti, whole wheat
Brown beans	Lentils	Strawberries
Brown rice, steamed	Lima beans	Tomato juice
Buckwheat	Mango	Tomatoes
Butterbeans	Mushrooms	Wheat, whole grain
Buttermilk		

Moderate Glycemic Index Foods

Angel food cake	Lentil soup	Semolina
Bran Chex cereal	Life cereal	Special K cereal
Buckwheat	Linguine	Stoned Wheat Thins
Chocolate	Macaroni	Sweet potatoes
Corn chips	Pineapple, fresh	Taco shells
Cornmeal	Pizza, cheese, regular crust	Taro
Couscous	Puffed wheat cereal	Tortilla chips
Croissants	Raisins	Wheat Thins
Instant noodles	Rice	Yams
Kiwis		

High Glycemic Index Foods

Bagels	Graham crackers	Rice cakes
Baguettes	Grape-Nuts cereal	Rice Chex cereal
Broad beans	Hamburger buns	Rice Krispies cereal
Carrots, fresh	High-fiber crisp rye bread	Rice pasta, brown
Cheerios cereal	Honey	Rye flour
Cocoa Puffs cereal	Kaiser rolls	Shortbread
Corn Chex cereal	Life Savers candy	Shredded Wheat cereal
Corn Flakes cereal	Macaroni and cheese, boxed	Soft drinks, regular
Cream of Wheat cereal, regular and instant	Melba toast	Tofu frozen dessert
Doughnuts	Popcorn	Vanilla wafers
English muffins	Potatoes, white (baked)	Waffles
French fries	Pumpkin	Watermelon
		Wheat bran cereal

Although it's vital to know the glycemic index of various foods when choosing a diet to treat insulin resistance, it's also important to keep glycemic load in mind. Glycemic load is a relatively new term that considers not only the glycemic index of a food but also the *amount* of carbohydrates found in that food. You see, if a food has a carbohydrate that converts quickly to glucose but the amount of that carbohydrate in the food is small, the food will have little impact on blood sugar and insulin levels. For example, in the table on page 157, you can see that carrots have a high GI ranking. However, because carrots are relatively low in carbs, you would have to eat a pound a day to raise your blood sugar and insulin levels. That's why carrots have a low GL of only about 5, and when it comes to GL, the lower the number, the better. A GL of 10 or less is considered low, a GL between 11 and 19 is medium, and a GL of 20 or more is considered high. If this sounds tricky, don't worry—both the GI and the GL of many foods have already been determined for you, making it easy to choose foods that will help keep blood glucose at a healthful level. One of the most complete books available is Shari Lieberman's *Glycemic Index Food Guide*, which lists the GI and GL of hundreds of foods and beverages.

Before we leave the subject of glycemic index and glycemic load, it's important to note that GI and GL rankings can actually be deceptive in the case of certain foods. Take ice cream, for example. Premium ice cream has a low GI and a low GL because its high fat content slows the rate at which it's digested, and therefore slows the rate at which it causes blood glucose levels to rise. But, as you know, all the fat and sugar found in this treat are sure to put on pounds. So besides looking at GI and GL, you'll want to choose unprocessed nutrient-rich foods like whole fruits, whole vegetables, and lean proteins. Always consider the entire food and not just its effect on blood glucose. Also be aware that by adding fiber to a meal, you can slow the rate at which the foods are converted to sugar, and consequently, also lower insulin levels. Fiber will also keep you feeling fuller longer—a plus when you're trying to lose weight. (To learn more about fiber and weight loss, see Chapter 3.)

In addition to modifying your diet, you can treat insulin resistance by using the appropriate nutritional supplements. The supplements listed in the table below can help lower blood sugar and make insulin work more effectively in your body.

SUPPLEMENTS TO TREAT INSULIN RESISTANCE		
Supplement	Dosage	Considerations
Alpha-lipoic acid	300 mg once a day	Improves blood sugar levels, so diabetics may be able to take less medication. If you have diabetes and are taking alpha-lipoic acid, check your blood sugar regularly.

Biotin	1 to 3 mg once a day.*	Use with caution if you have a duodenal or peptic ulcer and recurrent gastritis.
B-complex vitamins	Choose a B-complex vitamin that provides 10 to 50 mg each of vitamins B_1, B_2, B_3, B_5, and B_6; 200 to 400 mcg of folic acid; and 250 to 500 mcg of B_{12}. Take twice a day.	Speak to your health-care provider before taking if you have diabetes, liver problems, or anemia. B-complex vitamins may interact with certain antibiotics and anti-seizure medications. Whenever taking a B-complex vitamin, always take a multivitamin as well.
Bitter melon	1,000 mg one to two times a day.	Excessive doses may cause abdominal pain and diarrhea. Do not take if you are pregnant.
Chromium	1,200 mcg once a day.	Combining chromium with the protein picolinate allows your body to absorb the nutrient more efficiently. If you have kidney disease, consult your physician before taking chromium.
Cinnamon bark extract	100 mg once a day.	Cinnamon can lower your blood sugar. If you are taking a medication for blood sugar control, check your blood sugar levels and make adjustments as necessary. A lower dosage of medication may be needed.
Coenzyme Q_{10}	60 to 200 mg once a day. If you are using over 100 mg a day, take in divided doses.*	May reduce the effects of blood-thinning medication. May cause diarrhea in dosages above 100 mg once a day.
Copper	1 to 3 mg once a day.*	Your copper-to-zinc ratio is very important for your health. Whenever you are taking zinc, you must also take copper. Do not take copper if you have Wilson's disease. Also do not take the copper supplement form cupric oxide, which has a very low bioavailability.
Fenugreek	500 mg three times a day.	Can cause bloating, diarrhea, and/or indigestion. May cause urine to smell sweet. Do not take if you are on a blood-thinning medication.
Gymnema sylvestre	200 mg twice a day.	Can reduce blood sugar levels, so exercise caution if you are taking a medication that lowers blood sugar.

L-carnitine	500 to 1,000 mg once a day.*	Side effects are rare but can include agitation, headache, increased appetite, nausea, skin rashes, and vomiting. Ask your doctor before taking if you have kidney or liver disease.
Magnesium	400 to 800 mg once a day.*	Consult health-care provider for dosage if you have kidney disease. Discontinue use and see your doctor if you experience abdominal pain. Take a lower dose if it causes diarrhea. Magnesium's citrate, glycinate, gluconate, and lactate forms are more easily absorbed than its oxide form.
Manganese	2 to 5 mg once a day.*	If you have chronic liver disease, consult with a physician before taking.
Multivitamin, pharmaceutical-grade†	Follow the directions on the bottle.	Make sure to take only a pharmaceutical-grade multivitamin.
Omega-3 essential fatty acids EPA/DHA (fish oil)	1,000 to 3,000 mg once a day.*	In dosages above 4,000 mg, may cause the blood to thin. Do not take more than 4,000 mg a day if you are using a blood-thinning medication.
Taurine	500 to 1,000 mg once a day.*	Take between meals. Do not take with aspirin or any salicylate. Check with your health-care provider before taking taurine if you have kidney disease. Discontinue use if you suddenly have feelings of chest or throat tightness or if you break out in hives.
Vanadium	20 to 50 mg once a day.*	Do not take more than 50 mg a day.
Vitamin C	1,000 mg once a day.	Doses higher than 5,000 mg may cause diarrhea. Mineral ascorbates and Ester-C are buffered forms of vitamin C that lower the chance of diarrhea. Do not take high doses if you are prone to kidney stones or gout.
Vitamin D	To determine proper dosage, have your doctor measure your vitamin D levels. The minimum dose prescribed should be 400 IU.	In excessive amounts, vitamin D can be toxic. Do not exceed the dose prescribed by your physician.
Vitamin E	100 to 400 IU a day.*	Do not take with ferrous sulfate iron supplements, which destroy vitamin E. Do not take if you are on a blood-thinning medication. Take mixed tocopherols, the more active type of vitamin E.

Zinc	25 mg once a day.	The best-absorbed zinc supplements are zinc picolinate and zinc citrate. Side effects of zinc supplements may include nausea, stomach upset, and heartburn. If these effects persist or worsen, notify your doctor promptly.

*To choose an appropriate dose, see page 199 for information on dosage ranges.
† See page 197 for information on pharmaceutical-grade supplements.

Finally, you can help treat insulin resistance by making a couple of lifestyle changes that are not related to diet. Psychological stress has actually been found to increase glucose and insulin levels, so you'll want to incorporate some stress-reduction techniques into your daily life. Also, consider adding a healthy dose of exercise, which can improve your insulin and glucose levels and help you burn off excess calories. (See Chapter 6 to learn about stress and Chapter 2 to explore the importance of exercise.)

CONCLUSION

If insulin resistance is preventing you from shedding pounds, there is a lot you can do to improve your body's response to insulin and keep blood sugar levels under control. In many cases, dietary modifications and appropriate nutritional supplementation can treat this condition, enhance your overall health, and help you reach your desired weight.

On the other hand, insulin resistance may be just one of several factors that are keeping you from slimming down. If you take steps to correct this problem and still are unable to lose weight, be sure to explore the other chapters in this book, each of which examines a specific lifestyle issue, health problem, or biochemical factor that may be affecting your efforts to reduce. Once you have identified the contributing factors, turn to Chapter 20, "Putting It All Together," which will help you create an integrated weight-loss program that is suited to your needs.

17

Male Hormone Deficiency

Just about everyone has heard about menopause—the "change of life" that women experience between the ages of thirty-five and fifty-five, when hormone levels change. But did you know that men also experience a type of menopause? Sometimes referred to as *andropause* or *male menopause*, this is a slow process caused by a gradual decrease in the production of the male hormone testosterone. Much like women who experience a decrease in the hormone estrogen (see Chapter 14), men who produce lower-than-normal levels of testosterone can have a range of symptoms, with weight gain being one of the best known.

Although getting older is inevitable, gaining weight as a result of testosterone deficiency is not. Hormone replacement can help men feel (and look) better, regardless of their age or the reason for their lower testosterone levels. Moreover, lifestyle changes such as dietary modifications and exercise can boost metabolism even when hormone levels fall. This chapter will fill you in on the many functions that testosterone has in the body. It will then explore testosterone deficiency—why it occurs and how you can identify it. Finally it will explain how this problem can be relieved, allowing you to feel better and reach a healthy weight.

WHAT IS TESTOSTERONE?

Testosterone is the principal *androgen*, or male sex hormone. Baby boys begin producing testosterone in the womb—it's what determines their male gender—and continue to manufacture it in the testicles after birth, although levels remain low throughout childhood.

When boys reach puberty, generally between the ages of twelve and sixteen, the testicles begin producing more testosterone. The increased levels of this hormone further develop male reproductive tissues, such as the testicles and penis, and also lead to the appearance of secondary sexual characteristics, including increased muscle size, a deeper voice, and the growth of facial and underarm hair. Because muscle is such an efficient burner of fat, the added muscle mass—although it causes boys to "fill out"—helps limit the accumulation of body fat.

Levels of testosterone peak around the mid-twenties, although the "normal" range can be great—anywhere from about 270 to 1,070 nanograms per deciliter (ng/dL). As long as levels remain fairly high, this hormone can perform its many important functions in the body. Testosterone:

- Aids in mental concentration and cognition

- Decreases atherosclerosis (hardening of the arteries)

- Helps control blood pressure

- Helps control blood sugar levels

- Helps maintain a powerful immune system

- Helps manufacture bone

- Helps protect the brain against Alzheimer's disease

- Helps regulate cholesterol

- Improves mood

- Improves oxygen uptake throughout the body

- Plays a part in protein and muscle formation

- Reduces inflammation

- Stimulates and controls the development and function of the sex hormones and fuels sexual drive

WHAT ARE THE SYMPTOMS OF TESTOSTERONE DEFICIENCY?

As early as age thirty, levels of testosterone begin to decline very slowly—at the rate of about 1 to 1.5 percent a year. Studies have shown that more than a third of men age forty-five and over have low testosterone levels, which is often defined as 300 ng/dL or lower.

Although age is the most common cause of testosterone insufficiency, there can be other causes, including:

- Alcoholism

- Chronic kidney failure

- Cirrhosis of the liver

- Genetic problems such as Klinefelter's syndrome

- Hemochromatosis (excess iron in the body)

- Infection, injury, or loss of the testicles

- Inflammatory diseases

- Medications, especially hormones used to treat prostate cancer
- Pituitary gland dysfunction
- Radiation used to treat prostate cancer
- Stress

Whatever the reason for the lower testosterone levels, they do not always result in symptoms. When signs of testosterone deficiency do occur, they can include the following:

- Anxiety
- Backache, joint pains, or stiffness
- Decreased ability to deal with stress
- Decreased athletic performance
- Decreased bone density
- Decreased intensity of orgasms
- Depression
- Erectile dysfunction (inability to develop or maintain an erection)
- Fatigue
- High blood sugar levels
- High cholesterol levels
- Irritability
- Loss of body and facial hair
- Loss of memory or concentration
- Loss of muscle tone
- Loss of sex drive or libido
- Weight gain

If several of these symptoms sound familiar to you, perhaps testosterone deficiency is contributing to your weight-loss problem.

HOW DOES TESTOSTERONE DEFICIENCY CONTRIBUTE TO WEIGHT GAIN?

Earlier in this chapter, you learned that testosterone plays a role in the body's creation of muscle. That's why when boys reach puberty and experience a rise in testosterone levels, the size of their muscles generally increases, as well. Conversely, as levels of testosterone begin to fall—due to age or other factors—the body makes less muscle. This, in turn, lowers the rate at which the body burns calories, leading to the storage of more fat, especially in the abdomen. (Think of the "spare tire" that so many middle-aged men have around their waist.) But that's just a portion of the weight-gain story.

Although many people do not realize it, the male body also makes and circulates small amounts of the female hormone *estrogen,* which is needed for sperm development, strong bones, memory and focus, and many other important functions. In some cases, levels of testosterone get so low that they are unable to balance the effects of the estrogen. This

What Can Cause Higher Levels of Estrogen in Men?

As described on pages 166 to 167, the combination of aging and weight gain can lead to the production of higher levels of estrogen in the male body. But other factors, too, can have this effect, including alterations in liver function, zinc deficiency, the overuse of alcohol, and exposure to *xenoestrogens*— hormone-like substances found in external sources, such as commercially raised poultry and some industrially made compounds. In addition, certain medications have been found to elevate estrogen levels in men. Drugs with this potential effect include the following:

- Antacids, such as cimetidine (Tagamet) and omeprazole (Prilosec).

- Antibiotics, such as cefazolin, erythromycin, isoniazid (Laniazid, Nydrazid), ofloxacin, penicillin, sulfa drugs, and tetracycline.

- Antidepressants, such as fluoxitine (Prozac), fluvoxamine (Luvox), paroxetine (Paxil), and sertraline (Zoloft).

- Antifungal drugs that act as testosterone receptor inhibitors, such as fluconazole (Diflucan), itraconazole (Sporanox), ketoconazole (Nizoral), and miconazole (Monistat).

- Antipsychotics, such as haloperidol and thorazine.

- Cholesterol-lowering drugs, such as lovastatin (Mevacor), simvistatin (Zocor), and other statins.

- Drugs of abuse, including alcohol, amphetamines, cocaine, and marijuana.

- Heart and blood pressure medications, such as amiodarone (Cordarone), methyldopa (Aldomett), propranolol (Inderal), quinidine, and warfarin (Coumadin).

- Pain/anti-inflammatory drugs, such as NSAIDS—aspirin, ibuprofen (Advil, Motrin), and ketoprofen (Orudis)—and propoxeyphene (Darvon).

condition can lead to the accumulation of additional body fat. To make matters worse, fat produces an enzyme that is known as *aromatase,* which converts testosterone to estrogen, further throwing off the delicate balance of hormones and, ultimately, causing weight to spiral out of control.

HOW DO YOU DETERMINE IF YOU HAVE TESTOSTERONE DEFICIENCY?

Decreasing production of testosterone is a normal part of the aging process and should not be a cause for concern in the absence of medical problems. But if you have reason to believe that testosterone deficiency is behind your weight gain or is contributing to other health disorders, your doctor can order a standard blood test, a saliva test, or a urine test that will determine if your body is producing inadequate amounts of this androgen or problematic levels of estrogen. Testosterone levels fluctuate during the day, so many doctors prefer to run these tests in the morning, when testosterone levels are at their highest.

Be aware that different laboratories have different ways of defining what is a "normal" level of testosterone. Your doctor will use both the laboratory results and your medical history and symptoms to determine if your hormone levels may be causing trouble.

WHAT CAN YOU DO TO LOSE WEIGHT?

If tests have determined that you have testosterone deficiency, you can help your body lose weight—and potentially relieve other health problems—through testosterone replacement therapy. Replacement testosterone is available in a number of forms, including intramuscular injections, oral tablets, a testosterone patch that is applied to the body, and a testosterone gel that is rubbed into the skin. I recommend the gel, as it can be compounded in the exact dosage you need. Moreover, when testosterone deficiency has resulted in erectile dysfunction, transdermal (through the skin) testosterone is effective 81 percent of the time. Oral testosterone is effective only 51 percent of the time, and injections, only 53 percent of the time. Make sure that your doctor prescribes natural testosterone rather than a synthetic form of the hormone. (For more information about hormone replacement therapy, see the inset "Before Beginning Hormone Replacement" on page 142 of Chapter 14.)

Because testosterone is believed to fuel cancerous cells, men who have active prostate cancer or breast cancer should not use testosterone therapy. Screening for prostate cancer is a must before therapy is started.

In most cases, testosterone replacement therapy is safe, but it can result in the following side effects, particularly if you use testosterone when you really don't need it:

- Acne and/or oily skin
- Changes in cholesterol concentrations
- Flushing of the skin
- Increased body hair

- Increased red cell count
- Infertility
- Sleep apnea, a condition that disrupts breathing during sleep

If tests indicate that estrogen levels are too high, you can try taking supplements of copper, zinc, and low-dose vitamin E, which have been found to effectively decrease estrogen. (See the table below.) Weight loss may also be helpful. If these methods are not successful, your physician can prescribe anastrozole (Arimidex), a medication that reduces estrogen levels.

SUPPLEMENTS TO LOWER ESTROGEN IN MEN		
Supplement	Dosage	Considerations
Copper	1 to 3 mg once a day.*	Your copper-to-zinc ratio is very important for your health. Always take zinc if you are taking copper. Do not take copper if you have Wilson's disease. Also do not take the copper supplement cupric oxide, which has a very low bioavailability.
Vitamin E	100 to 400 IU a day.*	Do not take with ferrous sulfate iron supplements, which destroy vitamin E. Do not take if you are on a blood-thinning medication. Take mixed tocopherols, the more active type of vitamin E.
Zinc	25 mg once a day.	The best-absorbed zinc supplements are zinc picolinate and zinc citrate. Side effects of zinc supplements may include nausea, stomach upset, and heartburn. If these effects persist or worsen, notify your doctor promptly.

*To choose an appropriate dose, see page 199 for information on dosage ranges.

Estrogen can also be lowered through diet. To improve your testosterone-to-estrogen balance, try eating more cruciferous vegetables, like broccoli, Brussels sprouts, cauliflower, and kale, as well as oysters and other shellfish.

Finally, remember that hormonal problems don't have to lead to weight gain. Many men continue to eat as they did when they were in their twenties even after their metabolism has slowed down due to age. This, of course, leads to added weight because the body is simply unable to burn calories the way it did when testosterone levels were high. By limiting portion sizes, choosing healthier low-fat foods, and increasing physical activity, you will have greater success losing the pounds caused by a sluggish metabolism.

CONCLUSION

If hormone deficiency or imbalance is preventing you from shedding pounds, there is a lot you can do to improve your body's balance of these essential compounds. Dietary modifications, nutritional supplementation, exercise, and, when necessary, hormone replacement therapy can improve your overall health and allow you to reach your desired weight.

On the other hand, male hormone dysfunction may be just one of several factors that are keeping you from losing weight. If you take steps to treat hormonal problems and are still unable to shed extra pounds, be sure to explore the other chapters in this book, each of which examines a specific lifestyle issue, health problem, or biochemical factor that may be affecting your efforts to reduce. Once you have identified the contributing factors, turn to Chapter 20, "Putting It All Together," which will help you create an integrated weight-loss program that is suited to your needs.

18

Neurotransmitter Dysfunction

Are you feeling hungry? Are you craving salty chips or sweets? Or are you feeling full and satisfied? None of these sensations can be experienced without *neurotransmitters*—chemicals that allow messages to be sent from one part of the brain to another. When the body produces the correct amounts of these chemicals, your brain is in sync with your body. When you've had enough to eat, for instance, your brain tells you to stop. But when the levels of the various neurotransmitters are not right, and especially when levels are low, a variety of problems can occur, including the inability to feel that you are full and should stop eating. Because the brain is the command center of the body and tells the body what to feel and what to do, communication problems caused by neurotransmitter dysfunction can also cause other health problems—anxiety and depression, for example—some of which can lead to weight gain.

Although you may think that the production and use of neurotransmitters is out of your control, the fact is that a healthy diet as well as other important lifestyle components can help you maintain the brain chemicals you need. This, in turn, can protect your overall health, promote a feeling of well-being, and enable you to shed extra pounds.

WHAT ARE NEUROTRANSMITTERS?

The brain is composed of over 100 billion nerve cells called *neurons*. It is through the neurons that the brain passes on the information (or signals) that allow you to recognize and react physically and emotionally to both your internal thoughts and external stimuli such as heat and cold. Every time you respond to an event or a feeling, every time you feel happy or sad, hungry or full, it is because of this system of message transmission. Neurons even send the physiological messages that enable your body to regulate blood pressure, blood sugar levels, and other important body processes.

Since neurons don't touch each other physically, but are separated by gaps called *synapses,* the messages (which are electrochemical signals) cannot move directly from one neuron to another. Instead, chemical neurotransmitters bridge the gaps, passing on the information from cell to cell. This happens very quickly, with millions of neurons being affected in an instant.

The brain produces two basic types of neurotransmitters. *Excitatory neurotransmitters* promote the transmission of information from one neuron to another and have a stimulating effect on the body. They include aspartic acid, epinephrine (also known as adrenaline), glutamate, histamine, norepinephrine, and PEA (phenylethylamine). *Inhibitory neurotransmitters* decrease the ability to transmit messages and have a calming effect on the body. These chemicals include agmatine, GABA (gamma-aminobutyric acid), glycine, serotonin, and taurine. Dopamine is a unique neurotransmitter in that it is both inhibitory and excitory. Each of the substances just named regulates specific functions in the body. The table below fills you in on the major body processes that each chemical controls, presents common signs of deficiency, and lists the foods that can help your body produce adequate levels of each neurotransmitter. As you will see, these chemicals take part in every process in the body.

NEUROTRANSMITTER FUNCTION AND DEFICIENCY

Functions	Symptoms of Deficiency	Foods That Can Increase Levels in the Body	
Neurotransmitter: Agmatine			
• Aids wound healing	Agmatine deficiency is rare because the amino acid used in its manufacture is found in many foods and also made in the body.	• Avocados	• Meat
• Enhances immune function		• Beans	• Milk and milk products
• Enhances metabolism of fats		• Brewer's yeast	
• Helps build proteins		• Corn	• Nuts
• Helps produce glucagon and insulin		• Dark chocolate	• Oatmeal
• Increases circulation			• Onions
• Increases production of growth hormone		• Eggs	• Potatoes
• Increases sperm count		• Green vegetables such as asparagus, broccoli, peas, and spinach	• Raisins
• Inhibits accumulation of plaque in the arteries			• Seafood
• Needed for digestive health			• Seeds
• Reduces pain from poor circulation			• Soy
			• Whole grains

Neurotransmitter: Aspartic Acid		
• Aids energy production from carbohydrate metabolism • Assists production of DNA and RNA • Enhances immune system function • Helps protect liver from drug toxicity • Increases energy and endurance	• Depression • Fatigue • Reduced stamina	• Meat • Poultry • Seafood

Neurotransmitter: Dopamine		
• Controls the body's movements • Maintains good concentration, memory, and problem-solving • Provides feeling of enjoyment and pleasure, reinforcing certain behaviors • Regulates flow of information to other parts of the brain • Stabilizes brain activity	• Depression • Excessive sleeping • Inability to experience pleasure • Tendency to crave and eat junk food, especially sweets • Tendency to form addictions	• Almonds • Avocados • Bananas • Beans • Milk and milk products • Poultry, especially turkey • Pumpkin seeds • Seafood, especially salmon • Sesame seeds

Neurotransmitter: Epinephrine (Adrenaline)		
• Constricts arteries • Opens airways in lungs • Quickens heartbeat • Raises blood pressure • Regulates blood pressure • Regulates mental focus • Strengthens force of heart's contractions • Triggers release of glucose from energy stores	• Addison's disease • Allergies • Constipation • Decreased tolerance to cold • Depression or apathy • Fatigue • Low blood pressure • Low blood sugar • Muscle weakness • Need for excessive sleep • Poor circulation	• Beans • Eggs • Meat • Milk and milk products • Poultry • Seafood • Tofu

Neurotransmitter: GABA		
• Acts as muscle relaxant • Calms the brain • Lowers blood pressure • Prevents anxiety	• Anxiety • Insomnia • Rapid heartbeat • Seizures	• Beans • Fish • Brewer's yeast • Legumes • Dairy products • Meat • Eggs • Nuts

Functions	Symptoms of Deficiency	Foods That Can Increase Levels in the Body	
• Promotes secretion of growth hormone • Relieves stress	• Sensation that brain is racing out of control	• Seafood • Seeds	• Soy • Whole grains

Neurotransmitter: Glutamate		
• Balances blood sugar • Decreases food cravings • Enhances pain control • Enhances sensory perception • Fuels the immune system • Improves mental alertness • Increases energy • Maintains digestive health • Maintains muscle health • Neutralizes toxins • Plays a part in sensory perception • Promotes healing • Promotes healthy acid-alkaline balance • Promotes weight loss • Supports memory • Supports motor skills	Glutamate deficiency is rare because this substance is found in many foods and manufactured in the body.	• Beans • Brewer's yeast • Brown rice • Eggs • Fish • Meat • Milk and milk products • Nuts • Seafood • Seeds • Soy • Whole grains

Neurotransmitter: Glycine		
• Aids absorption of calcium • Aids in production of ATP, which stores energy within the cells • Calms aggression • Decreases sugar cravings • Helps build hemoglobin, proteins, DNA, and RNA • Helps detoxify heavy metals in the body • Helps maintain the nervous system • Needed to make bile acids • Needed to make glutathione, the body's most abundant natural antioxidant • Promotes healthy prostate gland function	Glycine deficiency is rare because this substance is found in many foods and manufactured in the body.	• Beans • Meat • Milk and milk products • Seafood

Neurotransmitter: Histamine		
• Plays role in development of organs • Regulates mood • Signals immune system to react to allergens, causing an inflammatory response	• Depression • Hallucination • Paranoia	• Citrus fruits, such as oranges and grapefruit • Garlic • Leafy green vegetables, such as spinach • Onions

Neurotransmitter: Norepinephrine		
• Enhances attention and focus • Constricts arteries • Increases blood flow to muscles and brain • Opens airways in lungs • Quickens heartbeat • Raises blood pressure • Regulates mental focus • Triggers release of glucose from energy stores	• Depression • Droopy eyelids • Fatigue	• Beans • Eggs • Meat • Milk and milk products • Poultry • Seafood • Tofu

Neurotransmitter: PEA (phenylethylamine)		
• Elevates mood • Enhances concentration • Increases energy • Promotes mental alertness	• Agitation • Confusion • Decreased alertness • Decreased sexual interest • Depression • Fatigue • Memory problems	• Bananas • Dark chocolate • Eggs • Milk and milk products Do not eat foods that increase PEA if you have PKU.

Neurotransmitter: Serotonin		
• Calms anxiety • Controls appetite and carbohydrate cravings • Regulates body temperature • Regulates sexual behavior • Regulates sleep cycles • Relieves depression	• Anxiety • Cravings for sugar • Depression • Fatigue • Insomnia • Loss of concentration • Poor impulse control	• Beef • Chickpeas • Dates • Eggs • Milk and milk products • Peanuts • Poultry • Seafood • Sunflower seeds

Functions	Symptoms of Deficiency	Foods That Can Increase Levels in the Body
	Neurotransmitter: Taurine	
• Aids glucose metabolism • Aids wound healing • Boosts immune function • Enhances use of calcium • Important for brain and nervous system function • Important for visual pathways • Improves insulin sensitivity • Improves liver and lung function • Lowers blood pressure • Lowers cholesterol • Prevents blood clots • Promotes kidney function • Stabilizes heart rhythms • Strengthens the heart muscle	• Anxiety • Depression • High blood pressure • Hyperactivity • Hypothyroidism (low thyroid function) • Impaired vision • Infertility • Kidney dysfunction • Seizures	• Brewer's yeast • Eggs • Fish • Meat • Milk and milk products • Seafood Avoid foods that contain MSG, since MSG degrades taurine.

It is important to understand that neurotransmitters aren't the only substances that help control body processes and emotions. Instead, as part of the body's highly complex chemical web, these substances interact with *hormones*—chemical substances that are produced by the body's glands. For instance, the stress hormone cortisol reduces anxiety by decreasing the release of the neurotransmitters epinephrine and norepinephrine. The hormone estrogen increases the concentration of the neurotransmitters serotonin, dopamine, and norepinephrine. It's impossible to describe all the interactions that take place in the body, but even this brief glimpse of the interplay between neurotransmitters and hormones highlights the fact that good health depends on the body's ability to maintain balance and coordinate the thousands of processes that occur on a daily basis. (To learn more about hormones, see Chapters 6, 10, 14, 16, and 17.)

WHAT ARE THE SYMPTOMS OF NEUROTRANSMITTER DYSFUNCTION?

Because neurotransmitters are involved in all body functions, and even play an important role in emotional well-being, there is a wide range of symptoms and disorders that can be caused by a deficiency or other dys-function of these chemicals. These problems include but are not limited to the following:

- Anxiety
- Attention deficit hyperactivity disorder (ADHD)
- Chronic muscle and joint pain
- Depression
- Excess weight
- Fatigue
- Fibromyalgia
- Food cravings
- Headaches and migraines
- Hostility
- Hypertension
- Inability to concentrate or focus
- Inappropriate hunger
- Insomnia and other sleep disturbances
- Irritability
- Irritable bowel syndrome (IBS)
- Obsessive compulsive behaviors
- Recurrent diarrhea or constipation

If several of these symptoms sound familiar to you, perhaps neuro-transmitter dysfunction may be a contributing factor to your weight-loss problem.

HOW DOES NEUROTRANSMITTER DYSFUNCTION CONTRIBUTE TO WEIGHT GAIN?

Research has shown that a number of neurotransmitters are essential in the control of body weight. When these neurotransmitters are in good supply, you feel full and satisfied after eating a healthful amount of nutri-tious foods. When these chemicals are depleted, however, it can take far more food to make you feel satisfied, and you may have frequent cravings for nutrient-poor, high-calorie foods such as sugary desserts. The result can be the addition of extra pounds.

Serotonin is believed to be the most important neurotransmitter in the control of weight. When serotonin levels are adequate, your appetite is controlled and you can resist sweets even when they are placed in front of you. In fact, when you have eaten a sufficient amount of carbohydrates, serotonin will actually send your brain a signal that tells it to stop eating carbs and begin eating foods that supply other nutrients. Eventually, the serotonin will signal your brain that you have had enough food, and you will stop eating until your body tells you that you are hungry again. When serotonin levels are low, however, the story is very different. Your brain will be unable to control your appetite, and you will end up overeating and craving refined-carbohydrate foods such as pasta, bread, cakes, and cookies.

As the table on pages 172 to 176 show, however, serotonin is not the only neurotransmitter that is directly involved in appetite control. Both glutamate and glycine control food cravings, and when levels of these brain chemicals are low, your appetite may increase. Other neurotransmitters play a less obvious but still important role in regulating appetite and weight. For example, dopamine and epinephrine both protect emotional well-being and fight depression. Since depression has been found to lead to weight gain (see Chapter 13 for more information), inadequate amounts of these brain chemicals can also lead to excess pounds. In fact, your body needs the proper balance of *all* neurotransmitters to maintain wellness and a healthy weight.

Can levels of neurotransmitters be too high? They can. The table below shows common problems that can be caused by abnormal levels of neurotransmitters, including overly high levels. Any of these disorders can result in excessive amounts of weight. (See Chapter 6, Chapter 13, and Chapter 5 to learn about the relationship between weight gain and stress, depression, and sleep disorders, respectively.)

HEALTH DISORDERS CAUSED BY ABNORMAL NEUROTRANSMITTER PATTERNS	
Health Disorder	**Neurotransmitter Pattern**
Abnormal Stress Levels	• High epinephrine • High histamine • High norepinephrine • High or low serotonin
Anxiety	• High aspartic acid • High epinephrine • High GABA • High glycine • Low agmatine
Depression	• High glutamate • Low agamatine • Low glutamate • Low histamine • Low norepinephrine • Low serotonin
Insomnia	• High epinephrine • High GABA • High glycine • High norepinephrine • High PEA • Low serotonin

HOW DO YOU DETERMINE IF YOU HAVE NEUROTRANSMITTER DYSFUNCTION?

If you are experiencing several of the symptoms of neurotransmitter dysfunction listed on page 177, or several of the deficiency symptoms included in the earlier table, you may suspect that you have unhealthy levels of one or more neurotransmitters. The only way to know for sure, however, is to visit a physician who specializes in metabolic and anti-aging medicine. (See page 211 of "Resources" for information on finding a specialist in this field.) This specialist can arrange for special urine tests that can detect neurotransmitters and their *metabolites*—the substances that result from the body's processing of each brain chemical. Although this testing is in its infancy, it can tell you if the observed range of each transmitter (the amount found in your body) is optimal, or if that brain chemical is being produced in inadequate or excessively high amounts. The practitioner who evaluates the test results should also be made aware of any symptoms you may be experiencing, such as insomnia, depression, and anxiety. All of this information is necessary to paint a complete picture of your health status and determine if steps should be taken to adjust your body's production of these important brain chemicals.

WHAT CAN YOU DO TO LOSE WEIGHT?

If poor levels of neurotransmitters are contributing to weight gain or your inability to lose weight, you'll be glad to know that there are steps you can take to restore proper levels of these vital chemicals.

The first step in correcting neurotransmitter problems is making sure that your diet supports a healthy level of these chemicals. The table found on pages 172 to 176 shows the foods that are particularly important in the production of neurotransmitters. Some foods actually provide the neurotransmitters themselves; beans, brewer's yeast, and a number of other foods, for instance, contain the brain chemical GABA. In other cases, the foods provide the basic chemicals needed for the body to synthesize that neurotransmitter. Serotonin, for instance, requires the amino acid tryptophan, which can be found in beef, poultry, and many other foods. By including these foods in your diet, you will go a long way toward helping your brain produce the chemicals it requires to stay healthy.

Another way to assist your body in neurotransmitter production is to get adequate exercise. Even short-term exercise has been shown to increase levels of serotonin and norepinephrine, both of which play an important part in appetite control. And, of course, exercise directly burns calories and steps up metabolism, boosting your efforts to lose weight. (To learn more about exercise and weight loss, see Chapter 2.)

If tests have determined that your levels of one or several neurotransmitters are very low, you may be able to take supplements that provide either the chemical itself or the chemical that your body requires to produce it. (Note that supplements are not available for all neurotransmitters.) The following table suggests dosages and presents considerations that you should keep in mind when taking these substances. Be sure to consult a metabolic and anti-aging specialist before using these supplements.

SUPPLEMENTS TO TREAT NEUROTRANSMITTER DYSFUNCTION

Supplement	Dosage	Considerations
Arginine (increases agmatine)	500 to 1,500 mg twice a day.*	Be aware that arginine can increase herpes simplex outbreaks in some people. If you are taking arginine long-term, consult a physician to see if you also need to take L-lysine.
5-HTP (5-hydroxy-tryptophan) (increases serotonin)	25 to 150 mg twice a day.*	Do not take 5-HTP if you are taking an SSRI, MAO inhibitor, or other antidepressant.
GABA (Gamma-aminobutyric acid)	• If you weigh less than 125 pounds, take 375 mg three times a day. • If you weigh more than 125 pounds, take 750 mg three times a day.	GABA may cause a tingling sensation in the face and slight shortness of breath; this should last for only a few minutes. GABA may make you drowsy, so take it in the evening. Do not take GABA if you have kidney or liver disease.
Glutamine (increases glutamate)	5 to 10 g once a day.*	If you have a sensitivity to monosodium glutamate (MSG), use glutamine with caution, as your body metabolizes glutamine into glutamate. If you are taking medications for seizures, use glutamine only under the direction of your doctor.
Glycine	250 to 1,500 mg twice a day.*	Do not take glycine if you are taking clozapine or another atypical anti-psychotic medication.

L-theanine (aids in the formation of GABA)	200 to 400 mg twice a day.*	Do not use if you are taking blood pressure medication or stimulant drugs. Women who are pregnant or breast-feeding should avoid use. L-theanine is intended for short-term use only.
Taurine	500 to 1,000 mg once a day.*	Take between meals. Do not take with aspirin or any salicylate. Check with your health-care provider before taking taurine if you have kidney disease. Discontinue use if you suddenly have feelings of chest or throat tightness or if you break out in hives.
Tryptophan, pharmaceutical grade† (increases serotonin)	Your physician must prescribe the appropriate dosage.	Make sure to take only pharmaceutical-grade tryptophan. Do not take if you are on an antidepressant. Do not take if you have kidney disease unless you are working with a physician.

*To choose an appropriate dose, see page 199 for information on dosage ranges.
† See page 197 for information on pharmaceutical-grade supplements.

CONCLUSION

If neurotransmitter dysfunction is preventing you from shedding pounds, there is a great deal you can do to improve your body's balance of these important chemicals. In many cases, dietary modifications and appropriate nutritional supplementation can treat this condition, improve your overall health, and help you reach your desired weight.

On the other hand, the inadequate production of neurotransmitters may be just one of several factors that are keeping you from shedding pounds. If you take steps to treat this disorder and still are unable to lose weight, be sure to explore the other chapters in this book, each of which examines a specific lifestyle issue, health problem, or biochemical factor that may be affecting your efforts to reduce. Once you have identified the contributing factors, turn to Chapter 20, "Putting It All Together," which will help you create an integrated weight-loss program that is suited to your needs.

19

Pregnenolone Insufficiency

Earlier in this book, you learned how hormones like progesterone, estrogen, and testosterone each play a role in helping the body achieve a healthy body weight, as well as performing many other important functions. What you may not know is that none of these hormones could exist without the substance known as *pregnenolone*. Pregnenolone has been called the "mother hormone" simply because it is used to make so many of the hormones that enable your body to function properly.

So far, so good. Your body uses pregnenolone—which is itself a hormone—to produce other hormones, and these compounds help keep you healthy. But there's a catch: Not everyone makes all the pregnenolone they need. In fact, some people make only about 65 percent of the amount required to keep the body on track. The result can be a myriad of health problems, including weight gain and difficulty in shedding extra pounds.

Fortunately, you can increase your body's level of pregnenolone. And by restoring sufficient amounts of this master hormone, you can enhance your level of wellness and achieve a better body weight.

WHAT IS PREGNENOLONE?

Pregnenolone is a naturally occurring substance and the *precursor* of all steroid hormones, which means that the body uses it to make cortisol, DHEA (dehydroepiandrosterone), estrogen, progesterone, and testosterone. The body produces pregnenolone both in the brain and in the adrenal glands, which are located on top of the kidneys. This important chemical compound is synthesized from cholesterol, which is a type of fat found primarily in meat and dairy products.

183

In addition to enabling the body to produce the steroid hormones, pregnenolone:

- Blocks the production of acid-forming compounds

- Elevates mood

- Enhances learning and memory

- Fights inflammation

- Helps repair nerve damage

- Improves energy, both physically and mentally

- Improves sleep

- Increases resistance to stress

- Reduces pain and inflammation

- Regulates the action of some neurotransmitters (see Chapter 18)

- Regulates the balance between excitation and inhibition in the nervous system

The body's production of pregnenolone peaks at about age thirty-five and then begins a long, slow decline. By the time you are seventy-five, your body is making 65 percent less pregnenolone than it did in your mid-thirties.

WHAT ARE THE SYMPTOMS OF PREGNENOLONE INSUFFICIENCY?

Inadequate amounts of pregnenolone can result from the aging process, high levels of stress, low levels of cholesterol, or hypothyroidism (an underactive thyroid). Because this substance is needed for the body's synthesis of several crucial hormones, low levels can lead to inadequate production of cortisol, DHEA, estrogen, progesterone, and testosterone. They are also associated with the following symptoms:

- Arthritis

- Cravings for sweets

- Depression

- Dry eyes

- Dry, thin skin

- Fatigue

- Inability to deal with stress
- Insomnia
- Lack of focus
- Loss of libido (sex drive)

- Low body temperature
- Memory problems
- Unexplained hair loss, especially in the pubic region and armpits

If several of these symptoms sound familiar to you, perhaps a low level of pregnenolone is contributing to your weight-loss problems.

HOW DOES PREGNENOLONE INSUFFICIENCY CONTRIBUTE TO WEIGHT GAIN?

Earlier in this chapter, you learned that because pregnenolone is one of the raw materials needed by the body to make steroid hormones like estrogen, progesterone, and testosterone, a deficiency of this chemical compound reduces production of these hormones. One of the results of this hormone reduction is weight gain.

In women who have gone through menopause, decreased production of the hormone estrogen is probably the most significant factor in body weight changes. As the ovaries produce less estrogen, the body looks for other sources of the hormone. Because fat cells can produce estrogen, the body works hard to convert the calories from food into fat. This not only increases weight but also throws off your balance of fat and muscle, and since fat doesn't burn calories the way muscle does, you put on even more unwanted pounds, especially around the middle. This is why 90 percent of postmenopausal women experience a weight gain of ten to fifteen pounds, as well as a change in body shape. (To learn more about estrogen and body weight, see Chapter 14.)

In men, lower levels of testosterone are often responsible for excess pounds. When testosterone levels are adequate, the hormone promotes the body's creation of lean muscle, which is an efficient burner of fat. When levels of testosterone drop, however—which happens during male menopause and can also happen during female menopause—muscle is lost, metabolism slows, and body fat starts to accumulate. (To learn more about testosterone and body weight, see Chapter 17.)

If you read Chapters 5 and 13, you know that fatigue and depression are both associated with weight gain. Because pregnenolone insufficiency can lead to both of these conditions, it can indirectly result in excess pounds and even obesity. Similarly, the inactivity that is a frequent consequence of arthritis—another possible symptom of pregnenolone loss—contributes to weight gain as well as to the loss of calorie-burning muscle.

HOW DO YOU DETERMINE IF YOU HAVE PREGNENOLONE INSUFFICIENCY?

If you are over the age of forty, you can be reasonably sure that your body is not producing all the pregnenolone you need for optimal wellness. However, it is important to have your level established before you begin pregnenolone therapy. I suggest that you visit a physician who specializes in metabolic and anti-aging medicine. (See page 211 of "Resources" for information on finding a specialist in this field.) This specialist can arrange for and interpret your pregnenolone-level test, and then prescribe a safe and effective treatment.

WHAT CAN YOU DO TO LOSE WEIGHT?

There are no known foods or supplements that can increase your body's production of pregnenolone, so if your levels are low, you should consider pregnenolone replacement therapy. In the United States, you can obtain pregnenolone without a prescription, but since this substance will cause your body to make greater amounts of powerful hormones such as estrogen, it's best to use pregnenolone pills or cream only under your doctor's direction so that you get precisely the amount you need. (Also read the inset "Before Beginning Hormone Replacement" on page 142 of Chapter 14.) If you take too much pregnenolone, you may experience the following symptoms:

- Acne
- Fluid retention
- Headache
- Heart racing (palpitations)
- Drowsiness
- Insomnia due to overstimulation
- Irritability, anger, and anxiety
- Muscle aches

If you are taking pregnenolone supplements and you suddenly begin experiencing one or more of the symptoms listed above, speak to your doctor about adjusting your dosage.

You may also be able to raise your pregnenolone levels by decreasing your stress—especially if you are under the age of fifty-five. See page 51 of Chapter 6 for some tips on relieving this common problem.

Finally, keep in mind that deficiencies of hormones such as pregnenolone do not have to lead to weight gain. With or without hormone replacement therapy, you can boost a sluggish metabolism by increasing your physical activity, and you can help your body lose excess pounds by choosing healthy low-fat foods and restricting portion size.

CONCLUSION

If insufficient pregnenolone is preventing you from losing weight, you can take steps to raise your levels of this important chemical compound and, in the process, restore normal production of the hormones DHEA, estrogen, progesterone, testosterone, and cortisol. This may boost your weight-loss efforts while relieving other health disorders that could be affecting you.

On the other hand, pregnenolone insufficiency may be just one of several factors that are keeping you from shedding pounds. If you take steps to treat this disorder and still are unable to lose weight, be sure to explore the other chapters in this book, each of which examines a specific lifestyle issue, health problem, or biochemical factor that may be affecting your efforts to reduce. Once you have identified the contributing factors, turn to Chapter 20, "Putting It All Together," which will help you create an integrated weight-loss program that is suited to your needs.

PART IV

Solutions

Introduction
to Part IV

I n the earlier chapters of this book, you learned about many different lifestyle and physiological factors that may be making it difficult for you to lose weight. By now you may have targeted one or more lifestyle problems, such as lack of exercise or inadequate sleep, that are hindering your weight-loss efforts. Or perhaps you suspect that your difficulty is rooted in a health disorder such as hormone imbalance or insulin resistance. Whatever your conclusion, you are ready to take the next step toward a healthier, slimmer body.

Regardless of your underlying problem or condition, you will probably need to modify your diet and introduce some form of exercise into your daily routine. Without dietary modification and exercise, weight loss is virtually impossible. This chapter will guide you in following a weight-loss plan of your choice and in developing an exercise program. It will also help you choose the nutrient supplements that, in many cases, are key to resolving any underlying condition, and will tell you a little about the professionals who can provide further information, guidance, and support. The goal is to help you create an easy-to-follow, custom-designed plan that will improve your overall health while assisting your weight-loss goals.

20

Putting It All Together

Perhaps your weight-loss efforts are being hampered by a lifestyle problem, or, perhaps, by a health disorder. Whatever the underlying cause of your difficulty, you will most likely have to modify your diet and introduce exercise into your weekly routine if you are going to enjoy weight-loss success. The following pages provide helpful information that will guide and support you as you make these important changes. In addition, this chapter offers valuable advice on choosing and using the nutritional supplements that can help you relieve specific disorders and restore overall health.

DIETARY MODIFICATION

Many people believe that weight loss is simply an issue of calories in versus calories out—in other words, a balance between how many calories you eat and how many you burn up, implying that as long as you burn more calories than you eat, you will lose weight. While there is truth in this statement, it is also an oversimplification. The fact is that there are many variables, including genetic predisposition and metabolic rate, that can determine how easy or difficult it will be for you to lose weight. In fact, almost all of us know at least one person who seems to be able to eat as much as she wants without putting on excess pounds. If you've read the earlier chapters in this book, you know some of the reasons this happens, but the bottom line is that even if your metabolism is being slowed by inadequate thyroid hormone levels—and even if these levels can be improved through treatments that speed up your sluggish metabolism—you will ultimately have to lose weight the old-fashioned way, by watching your diet and getting enough exercise.

Earlier in the book, you learned about specific diet plans that can help you treat specific health disorders. For instance, in Chapter 9, you discovered how a Mediterranean-style diet can help you end the vicious cycle of chronic inflammation and weight gain, and in Chapter 16, you learned how a diet that emphasizes foods low on the glycemic index (GI) can help you prevent or treat insulin resistance. Whether you decide to implement one of these eating plans or you intend to simply limit portion sizes and focus on healthier foods, you may find that it is difficult to follow a plan without some outside guidance and support. If so, below, you'll learn about a variety of options that can help you choose a proven diet and stick with it.

Computer Support

The Internet is an extremely useful tool for research, information, and communication. If you want to learn more about low- and high-glycemic foods or you wish to explore Mediterranean eating plans, for instance, you can find a wealth of information through your computer. Just as important, the Internet provides several computer-based personal weight-loss websites that offer dietary support and guidance and help you self-monitor your program. You may decide on an option that involves a subscription fee, such as Weight Watchers Online, or you may prefer to use a cost-free service, such as the one that is provided by the government at www.mypyramid.gov. On the latter site, after you enter data such as height, weight, and gender, the site provides a general food group plan, a specific menu plan, and an online tool for tracking your diet quality and physical activity status. Links to nutrient and physical activity information are included.

If you have already selected a diet but feel that you would benefit from the support of other dieters, this, too, can be found on the Internet. Search for "weight-loss support groups," and you'll find several that can meet your needs while you remain in the comfort of your own home.

Consult with a Professional

Nutritionists, dieticians, bariatric physicians (doctors who specialize in obesity), and physicians who specialize in metabolic and anti-aging medicine can provide you with a personalized diet and weight-loss program. Just as important, regular visits to these professionals can help you stay on track with your program. In one study, results showed that weekly consultations with a nutritionist for one year helped people successfully lose weight and body fat. Moreover, metabolic and cardiovascular risk markers—such as waist circumference, blood pressure, serum triglycerides, and blood glucose—declined significantly for these patients. In other words, those dieters who work with a professional both lose weight and experience better health.

To find a nutritionist, a dietician, or a specialist in bariatric medicine or metabolic and anti-aging medicine, see page 211 of the "Resources" section.

Join a Weight-Loss Group Program

There are many weight-loss programs that offer both dietary guidance and in-person support. Two excellent programs are Overeaters Anonymous (OA) and Weight Watchers (WW). OA emphasizes the psychological and spiritual components of weight loss, with its central focus on commitment to the group. WW is also rooted in the fellowship of community, but is more focused on personal behavior. Both groups can help you successfully make important lifestyle changes, including the adoption of a healthier diet. Additionally, WW (along with some other popular programs) offers prepackaged meals that can be purchased either directly from the organization or in your local supermarket.

In a study conducted on dieters following the WW program, participants experienced positive psychological changes and improved quality of life. Furthermore, over the long-term, a large percentage of the people following Weight Watchers were able to successfully maintain their weight for a number of years.

While OA and WW are not the only weight-loss programs that offer support, these are certainly two that you may want to consider for yourself. A search of the Internet or your local phone directory will help you find an OA or WW group near you.

Personal Chef Services

For many people, finding the time to prepare and cook nutritious meals is a major roadblock when following a diet plan. Today, however, there are cooking services that will prepare meals and deliver them fresh to your home. These personal chef services are not always as expensive as one may think. In many cases, they prepare several complete meals in advance to your specifications, and put them in containers before delivery so that they are ready to eat at mealtime. Generally, the only time you need to factor in is that needed to heat up the dishes. To find a personal chef near you, see page 213 of the "Resources" section.

EXERCISE

The importance of exercise in weight loss is universally understood and accepted. If you have read Chapter 2, you know that exercise can boost your metabolism—not only during the exercise session, but throughout the day—so that your body is better able to burn calories and rid itself of excess fat. Exercise also improves overall health, helping you avoid or relieve a number of health disorders, from diabetes to heart disease to memory loss. In fact, for some problems, such as chronic inflammation (see Chapter 9), physical activity is considered one of the safest and most effective forms of treatment available.

Now that you understand the value of exercise in any weight-loss program, you can choose an activity that will help you burn fat both safely and effectively. Fortunately, to lose weight, you don't have to engage in brutal sessions at the gym. Something as simple as taking a brisk walk that lasts thirty to forty minutes, four or more times per week, can help you shed pounds. The exercises listed below, though, have been found to be particularly helpful in burning fat:

- Aerobics class
- Bike riding
- Brisk walking
- Jogging
- Roller skating/blading
- Swimming

When creating an exercise program for health and fitness, it can be beneficial to determine your target heart rate—the number of times your heart can safely beat per minute during an exercise session. For most healthy people, the American Heart Association recommends a target rate that ranges from 50 to 85 percent of your maximum heart rate, which is usually calculated as the number 220 minus your age. For instance, if you are thirty years of age, your maximum heart rate would be approximately 190 beats per minute (220 – 30 = 190). During exercise, your target heart rate could safely be anywhere from 95 (50 percent) to 162 (85 percent) beats per minute.

When starting your exercise program, aim at the lowest part of your target heart rate zone—50 percent. Then gradually build up to the higher part of your zone—85 percent. The closer you get to your maximum heart rate, the more calories you will burn during your exercise session. But keep in mind that *any* exercise will help boost your metabolism and maximize your health. If you find your heart beating faster than the 50-to-85-percent range, you should probably exercise at a slower, less strenuous pace and build your fitness level gradually.

How can you measure your heart rate? Immediately following exercise, place the index, second, and third fingers of one hand on the palm side of your other wrist, below the base of the thumb. Press lightly until you feel the blood pulse. Then, using a clock or watch with a second hand, count the number of times your heart beats within ten seconds. Multiply this number by six to get the number of beats per minute. If you have trouble taking your own pulse—and many people do—buy a heart rate monitor. Available in sports stores, these watch-shaped devices make it simple to check your pulse during physical activity.

As you know, every year, many people start exercise programs, and while some stick with it, others give up after a few days, weeks, or months. How can you maximize your chance of making exercise an integral part of a healthy lifestyle? The following tips can help ensure exercise success:

- Choose activities that are fun, and develop a repertoire of activities that you enjoy. That way, you won't get stuck in an exercise rut and give up due to boredom.

- Don't overdo it. Especially at first, choose low- to moderate-level exercises that will not exhaust you or cause injury. As you become more fit, slowly increase the duration and intensity of your activities.

- Wear comfortable, properly fitting footwear and loose-fitting clothing that's appropriate for both the activity and the weather.

- Find a convenient place and time for your workout. If there's a gym near your workplace, this might be a great place to exercise. If you have trouble budgeting time spent outside the house, try working exercise into your at-home morning or evening routine. Then exercise at about the same time each day, three to four times a week. If you make exercise a habit, you will be more likely to follow your routine.

- Exercise to lively music or while watching TV. This will make your workouts more interesting.

- Make exercise a social event by walking, running, or working out with a friend. This will not only make your physical activity less dull but also provide you with the emotional support and encouragement that you need to succeed.

- Be flexible and take advantage of different opportunities to exercise. Use the stairs instead of taking the elevator. Take a stroll in the mall while you're shopping. Park a little farther from your destination and complete the rest of the trip on foot.

While everyone can engage in some form of exercise, health concerns may make certain activities wrong for you. If you've been sedentary for a long time, if you are very overweight, or if you have a high risk of coronary heart disease or another chronic health problem, be sure to see your doctor for a full evaluation before beginning a physical activity program.

NUTRITIONAL SUPPLEMENTS

As you learned in previous chapters, the right nutrients—vitamins, minerals, amino acids, essential fatty acids, and other important substances—are key elements in weight loss. Nutrients are needed to manufacture the hormones and neurotransmitters (brain chemicals) that help regulate metabolism, to control blood glucose and insulin levels, to relieve inflammation, and to perform a host of other functions necessary for a healthy body. Moreover, every year, over 75 percent of your body—even your DNA—is replaced and reconstructed from the nutrients you eat or that you take in supplements. Because so many of the foods we eat are nutrient-poor—due to nutrient-poor soil, even whole fruits and vegetables may not be rich in the vitamins and minerals you need—supplements are necessary for a healthy body.

Not all supplements, however, are created equal; some are of higher quality than others. On the following page, you will first learn how to choose the highest-grade nutritional supplements. You will then learn how you can get the most out of the supplements you take.

Buying Supplements

The quality of the vitamins, minerals, and other supplements you buy will have a marked effect on the health of your body and, consequently, on your ability to lose weight. To begin, it's important to know that there are four grades of supplements. From highest-quality to lowest, they are as follows:

- **Pharmaceutical grade.** This grade meets the highest regulatory requirements for purity, dissolution (ability to dissolve), and absorption. Pharmaceutical grade supplements are 99-percent pure, with no binders, fillers, dyes, or other unknown substances. Quality is assured by an outside party—the United States Pharmacopeia (USP). This high quality does not come cheap, however. Pharmaceutical grade supplements can cost three times as much as supermarket supplements and are available only from compounding pharmacies, better health food stores, and doctors' offices. In some states, you need a prescription to obtain supplements of this quality.

- **Medical grade.** These supplements are also high in quality, but may not meet all the standards for purity set by the USP.

- **Cosmetic or nutritional grade.** Supplements of this grade are often not tested for purity, dissolution, or absorption, and may not contain the amount of active ingredients listed on the label.

- **Feed or agricultural grade.** Supplements of this grade are produced for veterinary purposes and should not be used by humans.

To experience the full benefits of your nutritional supplement program, choose pharmaceutical grade products when available. A good health food store usually stocks supplements of several different grades. Ask which ones are pharmaceutical quality. Generally, medical trials are performed using pharmaceutical grade supplements, and dosage recommendations are based on these high-quality products. If you use a product of a lower grade, you may be getting far less of the active ingredient than you need for good results. For instance, a pharmaceutical grade coenzyme Q_{10} supplement marked "100 mg" (milligrams) actually contains a full 100 mg of this nutrient. If you buy a lower-quality product, a capsule marked "100 mg" may contain only 25 mg of bioactive coenzyme Q_{10}, so you would have to take four times as much to receive the same benefits.

When buying nutritional supplements that are not of pharmaceutical grade, you still should purchase the highest quality that you can find. The following guidelines should help you identify the purest and most effective products available:

- Look for supplements that contain no preservatives or artificial coloring—nothing but the nutrient itself. Be especially careful to avoid ingredients and fillers to which you have a sensitivity or allergy. Usually, the supplement label will tell you if that product contains soybeans, dairy, gluten, and other ingredients that may be problematic.

- For greatest effectiveness, choose natural forms of nutrients—not synthetic forms. Natural vitamin E, for instance, is better absorbed and more active than synthetic vitamin E.

- Be aware that many herbal supplements have been found to contain contaminants such as arsenic, lead, mercury, cadmium, and pesticides. Look for herbs that have a seal of approval from the United States Pharmacopeia (USP), NSF International, or ConsumerLab.com. These groups test products for label accuracy, lack of contamination, and the ability to dissolve and be absorbed by the body.

- Make sure that the supplement is packaged in a container that protects it from the light. Amber-colored glass is the best choice. When you purchase the nutrient, ask if it requires refrigeration.

- Choose products that have been vacuum sealed to preserve freshness. When you puncture the paper seal over the container, you should hear a mild popping sound indicating that the vacuum has been broken. Also make sure that the container has a tamper-proof seal.

Using Your Supplements

The dosages of vitamins, minerals, and other nutritional supplements stated in the supplement tables found throughout this book are for adults who have normal kidney and liver function. For each problem addressed in this book, the recommended amounts are designed to give your body the nutrients needed to regain health. You will note that this amount is usually greater than the Reference Daily Intake (RDI), which is the quantity that the US government has determined to be sufficient for healthy individuals. The RDI does not promote optimum health and is not intended to help the body recover from specific disorders.

In some cases, I have recommended a dosage range instead of a specific amount. For instance, in the table on page 97 of Chapter 11, the dosage advised for magnesium is 400 to 800 mg. If you are working with a physician specializing in metabolic and anti-aging medicine, he or she will be able to prescribe the precise dosage for every nutrient you take. If you are establishing a nutrient program on your own, however, I suggest that you start with the lowest possible dose and maintain it for two weeks. If you suffer no side effects but do not experience any relief from your problem, increase the amount you are taking and split up the doses, taking one in the morning and one in the evening, for maximum absorption. (See the discussion below for more information on split doses.) If after two more weeks you experience no improvement, increase the dose again, never exceeding the upper dosage range. If the situation doesn't improve while taking the higher amount, discontinue use of the product.

For some supplements, the table advises you to split up the doses. For instance, the recommendation might be to take 200 mg of a vitamin or mineral twice a day (for a total of 400 mg). The body can absorb only so much of any nutrient at one time. By taking smaller amounts several times a day, you will maximize your body's absorption and use of that healing substance.

The third column of each supplement table lists "Considerations"—important facts about how the supplement should be chosen or taken, or how it may interact with other supplements and medications. Be sure to read these considerations before adding the supplement to your health regimen. (For more information about possible supplement interactions, see the discussion below.)

Understanding Supplement Interactions

The nutrients you consume through both diet and supplements will interact with the medications you take, the foods you eat, and the other supplements in your health plan. Unfortunately, some of these interactions can be detrimental to your health rather than beneficial. Before starting any supplement regimen, therefore, you must be aware of possible side effects or contraindications. The following discussions provide examples of problems that can occur from some fairly common interactions.

Combining Vitamins with Medication

Some medications can deplete your body of specific vitamins and minerals. Similarly, some vitamins can increase or decrease your body's absorption of some medications. The following list provides common examples of both possibilities. If you are on any of the medications named here, you must discuss any nutritional changes with your doctor or health-care professional. He or she will make sure your vitamins and medications do not interact and that any nutrients depleted through medication use are replaced.

- Long-term use of antacids can lead to decreased folic acid absorption.

- Regular use of aspirin decreases folate levels.

- Birth control pills and other forms of estrogen replacement deplete the body of B vitamins.

- Too much vitamin B_6 can decrease the effectiveness of levodopa (an effective treatment for Parkinson's disease).

The Effect of Food on Medications

Although this book discusses a variety of drug-free solutions to various health problems, it is possible that you are taking medications for the disorders discussed within these pages or for other health issues. If so, it's important to know that the food you eat interact with the medication you are taking. The following list explains how one particular food—grapefruit—can increase the risk of side effects from a wide variety of drugs and can make some medications less effective. This list is meant to illustrate that whenever you take a drug, you should discuss it with your doctor or pharmacist and read the package insert so that you are aware of how that medication can be affected by the foods you consume.

- Grapefruit can cause flushing, headaches, dizziness, and increased heart rate if eaten while taking calcium channel blockers (such as nifedipine, amlodipine, verapamil, and felodipine), which help decrease blood pressure.

- Grapefruit increases quinidine levels.

- Grapefruit can cause irregular heart rhythms if eaten while taking the antihistamine terfenadine.

- Grapefruit can increase levels of benzodiazepines (sedatives that include alprazolam, diazepam, midazolam, and triazolam).

- Antiarrhythmic medications, such as disopyramide (including Norpace) and quinidine sulfate, can cause magnesium deficiency.

- Colchicine reduces the absorption of beta-carotene. It may also reduce the absorption of magnesium, potassium, and vitamin B_{12}.

- Methotrexate, used to treat cancer and autoimmune disorders, can decrease beta-carotene, folic acid, and vitamin B_{12}.

- Estrogen replacement increases calcium absorption.

- Anticonvulsants (seizure medication) can deplete the body of carnitine and vitamin D.

- Histamine-2 receptor antagonists (H2-blockers), such as cimetidine, can prevent or block the production of stomach acid and decrease vitamin D activity.

- Grapefruit can cause kidney and liver toxicity if eaten while taking cyclosporine.

- Grapefruit can decrease the absorption of macrolide antibiotics such as clarithromycin.

- Grapefruit can decrease the absorption of the popular antihistamine fexofenadine.

- Grapefruit can increase the medication level of HMG-CoA reductase inhibitors (statin drugs).

- Grapefruit can increase the level of warfarin, a medication that affects blood clotting.

- Grapefruit can delay the absorption of Viagra, a medication used to treat erectile dysfunction.

- Grapefruit can cause hives if taken with the pain reliever naproxen.

- Grapefruit can lead to nausea, tremors, drowsiness, dizziness, or agitation if eaten while taking carbamazepine.

- Grapefruit can elevate blood levels and cause nausea, drowsiness, tremors, or agitation if eaten while taking amiodarone.

- Grapefruit can increase estrogen levels in both men and women. No interaction with medication is necessary for this to occur.

- HMG-CoA reductase inhibitors (statin drugs), used to lower cholesterol, stop your body from making adequate amounts of coenzyme Q_{10}.

- Medications to lower blood sugar, such as glyburide (including Diabeta), acetohexamide (including Dymelor), and tolazamide (including Tolinase), can lead to coenzyme Q_{10} deficiency.

- Digoxin (a medication usually prescribed for heart-related problems) can increase the rate of calcium excretion from the body.

- Fiber can decrease the absorption of digoxin.

- Diuretics (water pills) decrease magnesium, potassium, sodium, and zinc levels.

- Potassium-sparing diuretics deplete your body of folic acid, calcium, and zinc.

- Calcium can decrease the absorption of beta blockers.

Combining Vitamins and Minerals

When different vitamin and mineral supplements are taken together as part of a health regimen, they can interact with each other and affect the way in which your body absorbs and uses the nutrients. The following list includes a few examples of these interactions. The supplement recommendations presented throughout this book take these physiological responses into account and are balanced to work well within your body.

- Vitamin C enables your body to use selenium effectively.

- Vitamin C can enhance the availability of vitamin A.

- Too much zinc can decrease calcium absorption.

- Vitamin D increases the absorption of calcium and magnesium.

- Vitamin D helps your body use zinc effectively.

- Too much copper can decrease the uptake of manganese in your system.

- A vitamin A deficiency can decrease iron utilization.

- Too much iron can lower your manganese and copper levels.

- Too much vitamin B_2 (riboflavin) can cause a magnesium deficiency.

- Vitamin B_6 (pyridoxine) can cause a decrease in copper absorption.

- A vitamin B_6 deficiency can lead to a decreased use of selenium.

- A vitamin E deficiency can decrease absorption of vitamin A.

- Adequate phosphorus intake is needed to maintain vitamin D.

IF YOUR WEIGHT-LOSS PROGRAM DOESN'T WORK

If you are severely overweight, have tried relieving any underlying conditions that may be hindering your ability to lose weight, and are still unable to shed pounds, do not despair. Sometimes, physical or emotional issues can make it difficult or impossible to follow even a well-designed weight-loss program. Because excess weight can lead to so many serious health problems, consider consulting a bariatric surgeon to see if you are a candidate for weight-loss surgery. Visit the website of the American Society for Metabolic & Bariatric Surgery (ASMBS) to learn more about this option and to find a qualified surgeon in your area. (See page 212 of "Resources.")

My hope is that this chapter has guided you in creating an integrated weight-loss program that includes dietary modifications, appropriate exercise, nutritional supplementation, and, if necessary, professional assistance. I think you will find that good lifestyle choices can help relieve many of your health disorders and, in the process, enable you to shed excess pounds. You *can* make a difference in your life. This book will help you take the first steps toward greater health.

Conclusion

Unlike most other diet books, which focus on what the author hopes will be the next big fad, this book is designed for people who want to identify the underlying problems that have been hindering their efforts to lose weight. Your appetite and your body's ability to burn fat are regulated by a host of body chemicals and physiological processes. If any of these factors is amiss—for instance, if your thyroid isn't producing enough thyroid hormone—you are likely to put on weight that can be very difficult to lose. Similarly, poor lifestyle habits—such as getting insufficient sleep or consuming inadequate amounts of water—can cause you to eat more than you should eat, to crave the wrong foods, and to experience difficulty in shedding pounds. It's important to note, too, that these problems generally don't exist in isolation, but are interrelated and can result in a vicious cycle. For example, insufficient sleep can cause food cravings, resulting in the consumption of too many sweets. This, in turn, can lead to the medical condition known as insulin resistance, which further heightens the desire to eat more food.

With that being said, it is important to recognize that we live in a society that promotes both overeating and consumption of the wrong foods—most significantly, high-sugar foods that quickly raise blood glucose levels and contribute to the accumulation of body fat. You may need more than willpower to lose weight; you may also have to take supplements or medication to resolve medical issues. But even if you restore normal levels of hormones and other important body chemicals, you will probably still have to improve your diet and, ideally, increase your physical activity. It is very difficult, if not impossible, to reach and maintain a healthy weight on a poor diet. Don't beat yourself up if you occasionally "fall off the wagon" and indulge in a less-than-healthy food, but do limit your consumption of foods that can lead to weight gain. What I suggest—what

I do myself—is that after you achieve your weight goal, choose one night a week on which you enjoy your favorite treat. This will help keep you satisfied while maintaining healthy body function and weight.

If you have read through the chapters in this book, you may have already identified one or more lifestyle habits or health disorders that are affecting your ability to lose weight. This is an important step, but it is only the first step in your journey. The rewards at the end of this journey, though, can be invaluable. By pinpointing potential problems and creating an integrated plan of diet, exercise, and nutritional supplements, you can enjoy not only a slimmer body, but also a healthier, happier, longer life. I wish you the best of luck!

Resources

Throughout this book, diagnostic tests and professional consultations are recommended to pinpoint medical problems. For many disorders, nutritional supplements are advised as part of an integrated treatment plan. This resource list was designed to help you find the best in each category. Below you'll learn about diagnostic laboratories, information organizations, and companies that provide high-quality nutritional supplements. (Be aware that many of these supplement companies will distribute products only to your health-care provider or compounding pharmacies.) You'll also find organizations that can guide you to qualified professionals in your area who specialize in natural health, nutrition, anti-aging and metabolic medicine, or the treatment of obesity and weight-related problems.

DIAGNOSTIC LABORATORIES

Age Diagnostic Laboratories
1341 West Fullerton Avenue,
  Suite 123
Chicago, IL 60614
Phone: (773) 528-8500
Website: www.adltests.com

ADL specializes in integrative and anti-aging medicine, and offers over one hundred hormone and genome tests using saliva, urine, blood, and hair. Assessments focus on finding underlying causes of gastrointestinal problems, nutritional deficiencies, metabolic irregularities, and improper functioning of the immune and endocrine systems. Self-testing kits and

instructions can be mailed directly to patients' homes, but may require additional payment if not ordered by a health-care provider.

Doctor's Data, Inc.
3755 Illinois Avenue
St. Charles, IL 60174
Phone: (800) 323-2784
Website: www.doctorsdata.com

Doctor's Data provides testing for nutrient levels, gastrointestinal function, and environmental factors (such as drinking water) that may contribute to an individual's health problems. DDI tests can also be used to check and treat patients for conditions such as heavy metal toxicity, liver detoxification, and abnormal metabolisms.

Genova Diagnostics

63 Zillicoa Street
Asheville, NC 28801
Phone: (800) 522-4762
Website: www.genovadiagnostics
   .com

Certified in a number of areas, including immunology, toxicology, and hematology, Genova Diagnostics offers tests for the detection of diseases such as adrenal fatigue, diabetes, fibromyalgia, hypothyroidism, and inflammatory bowel syndrome (IBS). Genova also specializes in salivary and urinary testing of hormone levels and their metabolites.

Metametrix Clinical Laboratory

3425 Corporate Way
Duluth, GA 30096
Phone: (800) 221-4640
Website: www.metametrix.com

Metametrix specializes in nutritional, toxicant, and gastrointestinal function assessments, and offers other tests for stress indicators and immune function. These tests are used to identify nutritional deficiencies, toxicities, and metabolic abnormalities, as well as genetic and environmental factors that may be at the root of chronic health issues.

NeuroScience, Inc.

373 280th Street
Osceola, WI 54020
Phone: (715) 755-3995
Website: www.neurorelief.com

NeuroScience offers saliva testing to measure hormone levels as well as urine tests that can detect neurotransmitter dysfunction. Depending on test results, patients can choose to start a Targeted Amino Acid Therapy program (TAATP) to restore their hormonal and/or neurotransmitter balance.

Pathway Genomics Corporation

4045 Sorrento Valley Boulevard
San Diego, CA 92121
Phone: (877) 505-7374
Website: www.pathway.com

Pathway Genomics Corporation is a federally-certified and California State-licensed facility that offers genetic testing for a wide range of conditions and genetic markers. Your health-care provider will supply you with the company's saliva-testing kit, which you will use and then return. When all your results are ready, your provider will contact you and present a comprehensive easy-to-understand report of your DNA analysis.

Spectracell Laboratories, Inc.

10401 Town Park Drive
Houston, TX 77072
Phone: (800) 227-5227
Website: www.spectracell.com

This laboratory offers innovative testing in the areas of nutrition and cardiovascular function, in addition to providing a number of specialty tests for genotyping, aging, and omega-3 levels.

ZRT Laboratory

1815 NW 169th Place, Suite 5050
Beaverton, OR 97006
Phone: (503) 466-2445
Website: www.zrtlab.com

ZRT provides blood, saliva, and iodine/dried urine tests, as well as combination testing for more comprehensive assessments. It specializes in testing for cardiovascular function, hormone imbalances, and vitamin D

deficiencies. In some states, tests can be ordered through the laboratory's website. In others, they must be ordered through a participating health-care provider. Check with the company for details.

DIETARY SUPPLEMENT INFORMATION ORGANIZATIONS

American Botanical Council (ABC)
6200 Manor Road
Austin, TX 78723
Phone: (800) 373-7105
Website: http://abc.herbalgram.org
The American Botanical Council promotes the responsible use of herbal medicine. This organization offers reference guides on common herbs and their medicinal uses, safety ratings, and possible side effects.

Council for Responsible Nutrition (CRN)
1828 L Street, Suite 510
Washington, DC 20036
Phone: (202) 204-7700
Website: www.crnusa.org
The Council for Responsible Nutrition is the primary trade association that represents dietary supplement manufacturers and ingredient suppliers. The CRN website makes available numerous fact sheets and reports on herbal, sports, vitamin, and mineral supplements, as well as general information about supplement benefits.

Dietary Supplement Information Bureau (DSIB)
Phone: (202) 204-4723
Website: www.supplementinfo.org
The Dietary Supplement Information Bureau advocates for the responsible use

of vitamins, minerals, herbs, and specialty supplements. DSIB provides facts on an extensive list of dietary supplements, and its website features articles on common misconceptions about supplements, newly discovered medicinal uses for various supplements, and choosing the right supplement for your particular health goal.

Linus Pauling Institute
Oregon State University
571 Weniger Hall
Corvallis, OR 97331
Phone: (541) 737-5075
Website: http://lpi.oregonstate.edu/infocenter/
The Institute publishes important information about how vitamins, minerals, herbs, and other micronutrients can affect metabolism, immune function, cardiovascular health, cancer, and stress response.

Natural Products Association (NPA)
1773 T Street, NW
Washington, DC 20009
Phone: (800) 966-6632
Website: www.npainfo.org
The Natural Products Association is the oldest nonprofit organization dedicated to the natural products industry. Its publications and reference materials, which can be viewed on the NPA website, pro-

vide important information about dietary supplements, including fact sheets and tips for use.

NSF International
PO Box 130140
789 N. Dixboro Road
Ann Arbor, MI 48113
Phone: (800) 673-8010
Website: www.nsf.org

The NSF serves public health and safety by implementing national standards for food, drinking water, air, and the environment. Its website provides helpful information for consumers, including a comprehensive list of products that have been certified by the NSF and a Dietary Supplement Fact Kit that answers common questions and explains supplement labels and regulations.

PHARMACEUTICAL-GRADE SUPPLEMENTS

Designs for Health
2 North Road
East Windsor, CT 06088
Phone: (800) 847-8302
Website:
    www.DesignsForHealth.com
Products include Inflammatone (to treat chronic inflammation) and FemGuard + Balance (for hormonal support). A wide selection of tablets, capsules, formulas, and extracts that promote a range of health and wellness goals are also available.

Douglas Laboratories
600 Boyce Road
Pittsburgh, PA 15205
Phone: (800) 245-4440
Website: www.douglaslabs.com
Ultra Preventive X (a multivitamin and mineral supplement), Adreno-Mend (for hormonal support), and PQQ Plus (for neurological health) are some of the popular products manufactured and sold by Douglas Laboratories. This company also offers "support packs" for a number of health concerns, including detoxification and weight management.

Life Extension
PO Box 407189
Fort Lauderdale, FL 33340
Phone: (800) 544-4440
Website: www.lef.org
This nonprofit organization's online store offers a wide variety of nutritional and hormonal supplements, minerals, vitamins, and herbs. Products include Optimized TryptoPure (for serotonin production), Super Omega-3, and DHEA tablets for hormonal support.

Metagenics
PO Box 1729
Gig Harbor, WA 98335
Phone: (800) 843-9660
Website: www.metagenics.com
Metagenics' focus is on treating common health conditions such as obesity, diabetes, heart disease, and high blood pressure. Products include CandiBactin (for yeast infections), Energenics (for thyroid support), Insinase (for high levels of insulin), UltraInflamX (nutritional support for inflammation-related disorders), and other supplements for optimal health.

Ortho Molecular Products
PO Box 1060
3017 Business Park Drive
Stevens Point, WI 54481
Phone: (800) 332-2351
Website: www.orthomolecular
  products.com

Products include Adapten-All (for adrenal support), Candicid Forte (for yeast infections), Inflamma-bLOX (for gastrointestinal problems), SereTone (for mood enhancement), and other products designed to support your body's biochemical systems.

Pain and Stress Center
Billie Sahley, PhD
5282 Medical Drive, Suite 160
San Antonio, TX 78229
Phone: (800) 669-2256
Website: www.painstresscenter.com

This organization specializes in neurotransmitter support, offering all-natural supplements to help with anxiety, stress, depression, and other mental health issues. Their products include Sleep Link (for insomnia and other sleep disorders), Mood Sync (to improve mood and memory), and Tyrosine 850, a natural antidepressant.

Professional Compounding Centers of America
9901 South Wilcrest Drive
Houston, TX 77099
Phone: (800) 331-2498
Website: www.pccarx.com

PCAA is a complete resource for compounding pharmacies that need chemicals, devices, equipment, training, and/or continuing education. The company also provides information for doctors and patients. To find a compounding pharmacy in your area, contact PCCA by phone or use its online "Find a Compounder" service.

PROFESSIONAL AND INFORMATION ORGANIZATIONS

American Academy of Anti-Aging Medicine (A4M)
1510 West Montana Street
Chicago, IL 60614
Phone: (888) 997-0112
Website: www.worldhealth.net

The American Academy of Anti-Aging Medicine serves as an advocate for the specialty of anti-aging medical science. Visit its worldhealth.net website and click on "Directories" to find a local physician who specializes in anti-aging and metabolic medicine.

American Clinical Board of Nutrition (ACBN)
6855 Browntown Road
Front Royal, VA 22630
Phone: (540) 635-8844
Website: www.acbn.org

The ACBN is a national accreditation agency that develops educational, clinical, and ethical standards for the practice of nutrition, and certifies the health-care providers that meet them. ACBN's website contains a directory of services, physicians, and other health professionals who offer quality nutritional treatment and counseling, and also lists nutritional products certified by the agency.

American Herbalists Guild
PO Box 230741
Boston, MA 02123
Phone: (857) 350-3128
Website: www.
    americanherbalistsguild.com

The American Herbalists Guild, a nonprofit and educational organization, represents herbalists who specialize in the medicinal use of plants. Check the website to learn more about the specific herbs that may be used to treat your health issue and to find a qualified herbalist in your area.

American Society for Metabolic & Bariatric Surgery (ASMBS)
100 SW 75th Street, Suite 201
Gainesville, FL 32607
Phone: (352) 331-4900
Website: www.asmbs.org

The ASMBS is dedicated to improving public health through the treatment of obesity and related diseases. Visit the society's website to find a list of member physicians who practice in your area.

American Society of Bariatric Physicians (ASBP)
2821 South Parker Road, Suite 625
Aurora, CO 80014
Phone: (303) 770-2526
Website: www.asbp.org

The ASBP is a professional association for physicians, nurse practitioners, and physician assistants who are focused on

the treatment and management of overweight and obese patients and their related conditions. The society's website can provide a list of bariatric doctors in your area of the country.

Institute for Functional Medicine (IFM)
4411 Point Fosdick Drive NW, Suite 305
PO Box 1697
Gig Harbor, WA 98335
Phone: (800) 228-0622
Website: www.functionalmedicine .org

IFM is committed to promoting the adoption of functional medicine—patient-centered care that addresses the interactions among genetic, environmental, and lifestyle factors. Visit its website and click on "Find a FM Practitioner" to locate practitioners in related disciplines.

Metabolic-Anti-Aging Specialist.com
Website: www.metabolic-anti-agingspecialist.com

This website includes a Practitioner Locator that provides lists of qualified specialists in metabolic/anti-aging medicine in your area.

MyPyramid.gov
Website: www.mypyramid.gov

Created by the United States Department of Agriculture, this interactive website provides nutrition information and helps you develop an eating plan that is tailored to your age, gender, weight, height, and level of physical activity.

National Association of Nutrition Professionals (NANP)
PO Box 1884
Rancho Cordova, CA 95741
Phone: (800) 342-8037
Website: www.nanp.org

The National Association of Nutrition Professionals represents holistically trained professionals who focus on individual needs and overall lifestyle rather than endorse nutritional products. The NANP website allows you to search for certified nutrition professionals by zip code, city, or keywords that describe your priorities and health goals.

United States Personal Chef Association (USPCA)
4801 Lang Avenue, Suite 110
Albuquerque, NM 87109
Phone: (800) 995-2138
Website: www.uspca.com

A personal chef can prepare meals that are geared for your individual needs and tastes, and then package and store them in your refrigerator and freezer, ready for heating and serving. Visit the website of the USPCA to use the association's search feature, which can locate a culinary professional by city and state, zip code, or telephone area code.

References

Chapter 2. Insufficient Exercise

Grimm, J, et al. "Interaction of physical activity and diet: implications for insulin-glucose dynamics." *Public Health Nutr* 1999; 2:363–368.

Horber, F, et al. "Effect of regular physical training on age-associated alteration of body composition in men." *Eur Jour Clin Invest* 1996; 26:279–285.

Hughes, V, et al. "Exercise increases muscle GLUT-4 levels and insulin action in subjects with impaired glucose tolerance." *Amer Jour Physiol* 1993; 264:E855–E862.

Ivy, J, et al. "Role of exercise training in the prevention and treatment of insulin resistance and non-insulin-dependent-diabetes mellitus." *Sports Med* 1997; 24:321–360.

Lehmann, R, et al. "Loss of abdominal fat and improvement of the cardiovascular risk profile by regular moderate exercise training in patients with NIDDM." *Diabetologia* 1995; 38:1313–1319.

"Prostaglandins, brown fat, and weight loss." *Med Hypoth* 1989; 28:13.

Summary Health Statistics for U.S. Adults, www.cdc.gov/nch/fastats/exercise.htm: National Health Interview Survey, 2009.

Walberg, J, et al. "Aerobic exercise and resistance weight-training during weight reduction. Implications for obese persons and athletes." *Sports Med* 1989; 7:343–356.

Chapter 3. Insufficient Fiber Intake

Anderson, J, et al. "Dietary fiber: diabetes and obesity." *Amer Jour Gasteroenterol* 1986; 81:898–906.

Anderson, J, et al. "High-fiber diets for diabetic and hypertriglyceridemic patients." *Can Med Assoc Jour* 1980; 123:975.

Burke, V, et al. "Dietary protein and soluble fiber reduce ambulatory blood pressure in treatment of hypertensives." *Hypertension* 2001; 38(4):821–826.

Houston, M. *What Your Doctor May Not Tell You About Hypertension.* New York: Warner Books, Inc, 2003.

Klatz, R, and Goldman, R. *7 Anti-Aging Secrets.* Chicago, IL: Elite Sports Medicine Publications, 1996.

Landin, K, et al. "Guar gum improves insulin sensitivity, blood lipids, blood pressure, and fibrinolysis in healthy men." *Amer Jour Clin Nutr* 1992; 56:1061–1065.

Rodriguez-Moran, M, et al. "Lipid and glucose-lowering efficacy of plantago psyllium in type II diabetes." *Jour Diabetes Complications* 1998; 12:273–278.

Sprecher, D, et al. "Efficacy of psyllium in reducing serum cholesterol levels in hypercholesterolemic patients on high-or-low-fat diets." *Ann Inter Med* 1993; 119:545–554.

Chapter 4. Food Addiction

Barnard, N. *Breaking the Food Seduction*. New York: St. Martin's Press, 2003.

Basciano, H, et al. "Fructose, insulin resistance, and metabolic dyslipidemia." *Nutr Metab* 2005; 291:5.

Beck-Nielsen, H, et al. "Impaired cellular insulin binding and insulin sensitivity induced by high-fructose feeding in normal subjects." *Amer Jour Clin Nutr* 1980; 33(2):273–278.

Bray, G, et al. "Consumption of high-fructose corn syrup in beverages may play a role in the epidemic of obesity." *Amer Jour of Clin Nutr* 2004; 79(4):537–543.

Cella, F, et al. "Effects of dietary restriction on serum leptin concentration in obese women." *Int Jour Obes* 1999; 23: 494–497.

Challem, J. *Stop Prediabetes Now*. Hoboken, New Jersey: John Wiley & Sons, 2007.

Chan, J, et al. "Dairy products, calcium, and prostate cancer risk in the Physicians' Health Study." *Amer Jour Clin Nutr* 2001; 74:549–554.

Choi, H, et al. "Soft drinks, fructose consumption, and the risk of gout in men: prospective cohort study." *BJM* 2008; 336(7639):309–312.

Di Tomaso, E, et al. "Brain cannabinoids in chocolate." *Nature* 1996; 382: 677–678.

Elliott, S, et al. "Fructose, weight gain, and the insulin resistance syndrome." *Amer Jour Clin Nutr* 2002; 76(5):911–922.

Flavin, D. "Metabolic danger of high-fructose corn syrup." *Life Extensions* 2008:69–77.

Gaby, A. "Adverse effects of dietary fructose." *Altern Med Rev* 2005; 10(4):294–306.

Gao, X, et al. "Intake of added sugar and sugar-sweetened drink and serum uric acid concentration in US men and women." *Hypertension* 2007; 50(2):306–312.

Hallfrisch, J, et al. "Effects of dietary fructose on plasma glucose and hormone responses in normal and hyperinsulinemic men." *Jour Nutr* 1983; 113(9):1819–1826.

Hak, A, et al. "Lifestyle and gout." *Curr Opin Rheumatol* 2008; 20(2):179–186.

Hsich, P, et al. "Functional interaction of AT1 and AT2 receptors in fructose-induced insulin resistance and hypertension in rats." *Metabolism* 2005; 54(2):157–164.

Johnson, R, et al. "Potential role of sugar (fructose) in the epidemic of hypertension, obesity, and the metabolic syndrome, diabetes, kidney disease, and cardiovascular disease." *Amer Jour Clin Nutr* 2007; 86(4):899–906.

Koehler, P, et al."High pressure liquid chromatographic analysis of tyramine, phenylethylamine and tryptamine in sausage, cheese, and chocolate." *Jour of Food Sci* 1978; 43:1245–1247.

Miller, A, et al. "Dietary fructose and the metabolic syndrome." *Curr Opin Gastroenterol* 2008; 24(2):204–209.

Quyang, X, et al. "Fructose consumption as a risk factor for non-alcoholic fatty liver disease." *Jour Hepatol* 2008; 48(6):993–999.

Shah, N, et al. "Effects of milk-derived bioactives: an overview." *Brit Jour Nutr* 2000; 84 (Suppl1):S3–S10.

Stahl, S, et al. "The psychopharmacology of sex, part 1: neurotransmitters and the 3 phases of the human sexual response." *Jour of Clin Psy* 2001; 62:80–81.

Taylor, E, et al. "Fructose conception and the risk of kidney stones." *Kidney Int* 2008; 73(2):207–212.

Thuy, S, et al. "Non alcoholic fatty liver disease in humans is associated with increased plasma endotoxin and plasminogen activator inhibitor 1 concentrations and with fructose intake." *Jour Nutr* 2008; 138(8):1452–1455.

Wang, G, et al. "Brain dopamine and obesity." *Lancet* 2001; 357: 354–357.

Chapter 5. Sleep Deprivation

Andretic, R, et al. "Genetics of sleep." *Annual Review of Genetics* 2008; 42:361–388.

Banks, S, et al. "Behavioral and physiological consequences of sleep restriction." *Journal of Clinical Sleep Medicine* 2007; 3(5):519–528.

Benarroch, E. "Suprachiasmatic nucleus and melatonin: reciprocal interactions and clinical correlations." *Neurology* 2008; 71:594–598.

Bland, J. "Obesity and Endocrine Signaling." *Improving Intercellular Communication in Managing Chronic Illness*. Gig Harbor, WA: HealthComm International, Inc, 1999.

Brandenberger, G, et al. "Effect of sleep deprivation on overall 24 hour growth-hormone secretion." *Lancet* 2000; 356(9230):1408.

Brzezinski, A, et al. "Melatonin in humans." *New England Journal of Medicine* 1997; 336(3):186-195.

Chesson, A, et al. "Current trends in the management of insomnia." *Emergency Medicine* 2002; 34:11–20.

Edling, C, et al. "Occupational exposure to organic solvents as a cause of sleep apnea." *British Journal of Industrial Medicine* 1993; 50:276–279.

Foss-Morgan, R. *Hormone Replacement Therapy*. Haddonfield, NJ: Anti-Aging and Longevity Medical Center of Haddonfield, 2000.

Franzen, P, et al. "Sleep disturbances and depression: risk relationships for subsequent depression and therapeutic implications." *Dialogues in Clinical Neuroscience* 2008; 10:473–481.

Garfinkel, D, et al. "Improvement of sleep quality in elderly people by controlled-release melatonin." *Lancet* 1995; 346(8974):541–544.

Goldman, R, and Klatz, R. *Sleep for Optimal Health*. Chicago, IL: American Academy of Anti-Aging Medicine, 2003.

Haimov, I, et al. "Melatonin replacement therapy of elderly insomnia." *Sleep* 1995; 18(7):598–603.

Hastings, M, et al. "A clockwork web: circadian timing in brain and periphery in health and disease." *Nature Reviews Neuroscience* 2003; 4:649.

Herzog, E. "Neurosis and networks in daily rhythms." *Nat Rev Neurosci* 2007; 8:790.

Hobson, J, et al. "The cognitive neuroscience of sleep: neuronal systems, consciousness and learning." *Nat Rev Neurosci* 2003; 3:679–693.

Hornyak, M, et al. "Magnesium therapy for periodic leg movements-related insomnia and restless legs syndrome: an open pilot study." *Sleep* 1998; 21:501–505.

Imeri, L, et al. "How (and why) the immune system makes us sleep." *Nat Rev Neurosci* 2009; 10:199–210.

James, S, et al. "Melatonin administration in insomnia." *Neuropsychopharmacology* 1990; 3(1):19–23.

Krueger, J, et al. "Sleep as a fundamental property of neuronal assemblies." *Nat Rev Neurosci* 2008; 9:910–919.

LaValle, J. "Current concepts in metabolic regulation: the role of nutrients and novel agents." Detroit, MI: Module IV, Fellowship in Anti-Aging, Regenerative, and Functional Medicine, 2006.

Lieberman, S. *The Real Vitamin and Mineral Book*. New York: Avery Publishing, 1997.

Morin, C. "Psychological and behavioral treatment of insomnia: update of the recent evidence (1998-2004)." *Sleep* 2006; 29:1398–1414.

Nedeltcheva, A, et al. "Insufficient sleep undermines dietary efforts to reduce adiposity." *Annals of Internal Medicine* 2010; 153:435–444.

Nurnberger, J, et al. "Melatonin suppression by light in euthymic bipolar and unipolar patients." *Archives of General Psychiatry*, 2000; 57:572–579.

Nutt, D, et al. "Sleep disorders as core symptoms of depression." *Dialogues Clin Neurosci* 2008; 10:329–336.

Pace-Schott, E, et al. "The neurobiology of sleep: genetics, cellular physiology, and subcortical networks." *Nat Rev Neurosci* 2002; 3:592.

Pastora, J, et al. "Flavonoids from lemon balm (melissa officinalis l., lamiaceae)." *Acta Pol Pharm* 2002; 59(2):139–143.

Poeggeler, B, et al. "Melatonin—a highly potent endogenous radical scavenger and electron donor: new aspects of the oxidation chemistry of this indole accessed in vitro." *Annals of the New York Academy of Sciences* 1994; 738:419–421.

Schmidt, M. *Tired of Being Tired: Overcoming Chronic Fatigue and Low Energy*. Berkley, CA: Frog, Ltd, 1995.

Schutte-Rodin, S. "Clinical guideline for the evaluation and management of chronic insomnia in adults." *J Clin Sleep Med* 2008; 4:487–504.

Speroni, E, et al. "Neuropharmacologicial activity of extracts from Passiflora incarnate." *Planta Medica* 1988; 488–491.

Spiegel, K, et al. "Impact of sleep on metabolic function." *Lancet* 1999; 354(9188):1435–1439.

Spiegel, K, et al. "Leptin levels are dependent on sleep duration: relationships with sympatho-vagal balance, carbohydrate regulation, cortisol, and thyrotropin." *J Clin Endocrin Metab* 2004; 89(11):5762–5771.

Steiger, A, et al. "Effects of hormones on sleep." *Hormone Research* 1998; 49(3–4):125–130.

Tan, D, et al. "Melatonin: a potent endogeneous hydroxyl radical scavenger." *Endocrine* 1993; 1:57–60.

Vgontzas, A, et al. "Chronic insomnia is associated with nyctohemeral activation of the hypo-thalamic-pituitary-adrenal axis: clinical implications." *J Clin Endocrin Metab* 2001; 86(8): 3787–3794.

Vliet, E. *Women, Weight and Hormones*. New York: M. Evans & Co, 2001.

Willner, C. "Optimizing restorative sleep." Las Vegas: Module VIII, Anti-Aging and Regenerative Medicine Conference, 2010.

Chapter 6. Stress

Ahlgrimm, M. *The HRT Solution*. New York: Avery Publishing, 1999.

Barbieri, R, et al. "Cotinine and nicotine inhibit human fetal adrenal 11, beta-hydroxylase." *Jour Clin Endocrinol Metab* 1989; 69:1221–1224.

Barrett-Conner, E, et al. "A prospective study of dehydroepiandrosterone sulfate, mortality and cardiovascular disease." *NEJM* 1986; 37(9):1035.

Benson, H. *The Relaxation Response*. New York: Quill Publishers, 2001.

Bjomtop, P, et al. "Consolatory eating is not a myth. Stress-induced cortisol levels result in leptin-resistant obesity." *Lakartidningen* 2001; 98(48):5458–5461.

Bland, J. "Introduction to neuroendocrine disorders." *Functional Medicine Approaches to Endocrine Disturbances of Aging*. Gig Harbor, WA: The Institute for Functional Medicine, 2001.

Bland, J. "Normalizing HPA function." *Nutritional Endocrinology: Breakthrough Approaches for Improving Adrenal and Thyroid Function*. Gig Harbor, WA: The Institute for Functional Medicine, 2002.

Brownstein, D. *Overcoming Thyroid Disorders*. West Bloomfield, MI: Medical Alternatives Press, 2002.

Crayhon, R. "Aging well in the 21st century." *Seminar* 2002:24.

Darbinyan, VB, et al. "Rhodiola rosea in stress induced fatigue—a double-blind crossover study of a standardized extract SHR-J with a repeated low dose regimen on the mental performance of healthy physicians during night duty." *Phytomed* 2000; 7(5):365–371.

Epel, E, et al. "Can stress shape your body? Consistently greater stress-induced cortisol secretion among women with abdominal fat." *Psychosomatic Med* 2000; (62):623–632.

Fulder, S, et al. "Ginseng and the hypothalamic pituitary control of stress." *Amer Jour Chinese Med* IX (2):112–118.

Goldman, R. *Brain Fitness*. New York: Doubleday, 1999.

Gordon, G, et al. "Reduction of atherosclerosis by administration of dehydroepiandrosterone. A study of the hypercholesterolemic New Zealand white rabbit and aortic internal injury." *Jour Clin Invest* 1988; 82:712.

Grandi, A, et al. "A comparative pharmacological investigation of ashwagandha and ginseng." *Jour Ethnopharmacol* 1994; 44:131–135.

Heller, L. *The Essentials of Herbal Care Part II*. San Clemente, CA: Metagenics, Inc, 2000.

Kelly, G, et al. "Nutritional and botanical interventions to assist with the adaption to stress." *Altern Med Rev* 1999; 4(4):249–265.

Lieberman, S. *The Real Vitamin and Mineral Book*. New York: Avery Publishing, 1997.

Rege, N, et al. "Adaptogenic properties of six Rasuyana herbs used in ayurvedic medicine." *Phytotherapy Res* 1999; 13:275–292.

Stewart, P, et al. "Growth hormone, insulin-like growth factor-1 and the cortisol-cortisone shuttle." *Hormone Research* 2001; 56:1–6.

Tully, D, et al. "Modulation of steroid receptor-mediated gene expression by vitamin B6." *FASEB Jour* 1994; 8:343–349.

Vliet, E. *Women, Weight and Hormones*. New York: M. Evans & Co, 2001.

Wilson, J. *Adrenal Fatigue*. Petaluma, CA: Smart Publications, 2001.

Wilson, J. "Metabolic syndrome and adrenal fatigue: balancing the difficult patient." *BHRT for Female Patients Symposium*, Houston, TX, August 24–26, 2006.

Yeh, J, et al. "Nicotine and cotinine inhibit rat testes androgen biosynthesis in vitro," *Jour Steroid Biochem* 1989; 33(4A):627–630.

Zhu, U, et al. "The scientific rediscovery of an ancient Chinese herbal medicine: cordyceps sinensis." *Jour Alt Complem Med* 1998; 4(3):289–303.

Chapter 7. Insufficient Water Intake

Batmanghelidj, B. *Your Body's Many Cries for Water*. Vienna, VA: Global Health Solutions, 1992.

David, Y, et al. "Water intake and cancer prevention." *Jour of Clin Oncology* 2004; 22(2):383—385.

Chapter 8. Food Allergies

Appleton, N. *Stopping Inflammation: Relieving the Cause of Degenerative Diseases.* Garden City Park, NY: Square One Publishers, 2005.

Edwards, T, et al. "Failure to thrive." *Clinical and Environmental Allergy.* 1995; 25:16–19.

Gaby, A. "The role of hidden food allergy in chronic disease." *Alt Med Rev* 1998; 3(2):90–100.

Marshall, P, et al. "Effects of seasonal allergic rhinitis on fatigue levels and mood." *Psychosm Med* 2002; 64(4):684–691.

Rothenberg, M, et al. "A pathological function for exotoxin and eosinophils in eosinophilic gastrointestinal inflammation." *Nature Immunology* 2001; 2:353–360.

Chapter 9. Chronic Inflammation

Bland, J. *Clinical Nutrition: A Functional Approach.* Gig Harbor, WA: The Institute for Functional Medicine, 1999.

Blum, S, et al. "Effect of a Mediterranean meal on postprandial carotenoids, paramonase and c-reactive protein levels." *Ann Nutr Metabol* 2006; 0(1):20–24.

Bruunsgaard, H. "Physical activity and modulation of systemic low-level inflammation." *Jour Leukocyte Biol* 2005; 78:819–835.

Cesarri, M, et al. *Amer Jour Clin Nutr* 2005; 82:428–434.

Challem, J. *The Inflammation Syndrome.* Hoboken, NJ: John Wiley & Sons, 2003.

Colgan, M. *The New Nutrition.* Vancouver, BC, Canada: Apple Publishing, 1995.

Dietrich, M, et al. "The effect of weight loss on a stable biomarker of inflammation, c-reactive protein." *Nutrition Reviews* 2005; 63(1):22–28.

Erasmus, Udo. *Fats That Heal, Fats That Kill.* Burnaby, BC, Canada: Alive Books, 1993.

Esposito, K, et al. "Effect of a Mediterranean-style diet on endothelial dysfunction and markers of vascular inflammation in the metabolic syndrome. A randomized trial." *JAMA* 2004; 292(12):1440–1446.

Esposito, K, et al. *JAMA* 2003; 289:1799–1804.

Goodman, J. *The Omega Solution.* Roseville, CA: Prima Publishing, 2001.

Greenberg, A, et al. "Obesity and the role of adipose tissue in inflammation and metabolism." *Amer Jour Clin Nutr* 2006; 83(2):461S–465S.

Guilliams, T. "Managing chronic inflammation: natural solutions." *The Standard* 2006; 7(2):3.

Houston, M. "The metabolic syndrome: pathophysiology, diagnosis, clinical aspects, prevention and nonpharmacologic treatment: Emphasis on lifestyle modifications, nutrition, nutritional supplements, vitamins, minerals, antioxidants, weight management and exercise." *JANA* 2005; 8(2):28.

Lerman, R. "The essential fatty acids in psychiatric and neurological dysfunction." *Brain Biochemistry and Nutrition.* Gig Harbor, WA: The Institute for Functional Medicine, 2002.

Lerman, R. "Nutrients as biological response modifiers: fatty acids and inflammation." *Applying Functional Medicine in Clinical Practice.* Gig Harbor, WA: The Institute for Functional Medicine, 2002.

Lu, S, et al. "Relation between a diet with a high glycemic load and plasma concentrations of high sensitivity c-reactive protein in middle-aged women." *Amer Jour Clin Nutr* 2002; 75(3):492–498.

Miller, G, et al. "Chronic psychological stress and the regulation of pro-inflammatory cytokines: a glucocorticoid-resistance model." *Health Psychology* 2002; 21(6): 531–541.

Nicklas, B, et al. "Behavioral treatments for chronic systemic inflammation: effects of dietary weight loss and exercise training." *CMAJ* 2005; 72(9):1199–1204.

Qi, L, et al. "Whole-grain, bran, and cereal fiber intakes and markers of systemic inflammation in diabetic women." *Diabetes Care* 2006; 29(2):207–211.

Rakel, D, et al. "Inflammation: nutritional, botanical, and mind-body influences." *Southern Med Journ* 2005; 98(3):303–309.

Rountree, R. "Immune dysfunction and inflammation, Part II." *Applying Functional Medicine in Clinical Practice*. Gig Harbor, WA: The Institute for Functional Medicine, 2002.

Schmidt, M. *Brain-Building Nutrition: The Healing Power of Fats and Oils*. Berkeley, CA: Frog, Ltd, 2001.

Chapter 10. Thyroid Hormone Dysfunction

Adlin, V, et al. "Subclinical hypothyroidism: deciding when to treat." *Amer Fam Physician* 1998; 57(4):776–780.

Beard, J. "Impaired thermoregulation and thyroid function in iron deficiency anemia." *Amer Jour Clin Nutr* 1990; 52:813–819.

Berger, N, et al. "Influence of selenium supplementation on the post-traumatic alterations of the thyroid axis: A placebo-controlled trial." *Intensive Care Med* 2001; 27(1):91–100.

Berry, M, et al. "The role of selenium in thyroid hormone action." *Endocrine Rev* 1992; 13:207–220.

Brownstein, D. *The Miracle of Natural Hormones*. West Bloomfield, MI: Medical Alternatives Press, 1998.

Brownstein, D. *Overcoming Thyroid Disorders*. West Bloomfield, MI: Medical Alternatives Press, 2002.

Bunevicius, R, et al. "Effects of thyroxine as compared with thyroxine plus triiodothyronine in patients with hypothyroidism." *NEJM* 1994; 340(6):424–429.

Cavalieri, R, et al. "Effects of drugs on human thyroid hormone metabolism." *Thyroid Hormone Metabolism*. New York: Marcel Dekker, 1998.

Contempre, B, et al. "Effect of selenium supplementation on thyroid hormone metabolism in an iodine and selenium deficient population." *Clin Endocrinol* 1992; 36:579–583.

DeGroot, L, Ed. *Endocrinology*, Fifth Edition. Philadelphia: Elsevier Saunders, 2006.

Divi, R, et al. "Anti-thyroid isoflavones from soybean: isolation, characterization, and mechanism of action." *Biochem Pharmacol* 1997; 54(10):1087–1096.

Fed Register. 1997; 62(157).

Hale, A, et al. "Subclinical hypothyroidism is an independent risk factor for atherosclerosis and MI in elderly women: The Rotterdam study." *Ann Inter Med* 2000; 132:270–278.

Hertoghe, J, et al. "Thyroid insufficiency. Is thyroxine the only valuable drug?" *Jour of Nutr & Environ Med* 2001; 11:159–166.

Horst, C, et al. "Rapid stimulation of hepatic oxygen consumption by 3,5-di-iodo-1-thyrooninne." *Biochem Journ* 1989; 261:945–950.

Kohrle, J, et al. "The deiodinase family: selenoenzymes regulating thyroid hormone availability and action." *Cell Mol Life Sci* 2000; 57:1853–1863.

Lazarus, J, et al. "Lithium therapy and thyroid function: a long-term study." *Psychol Med* 1981; 11(1):85–92.

Lenon, D, et al. "Diet and exercise training effects on resting metabolic rate." *Int Jour Obesity* 1985; 9:39–47.

Meinhold, H, et al. "Effects of selenium and iodine deficiency on iodothyronine deiodinases in brain, thyroid and peripheral tissue." *JAMA* 1992; 19:8–12.

Nishida, M, et al. "Direct evidence for the presence of methylmercury bound in the thyroid and other organs obtained from mice given methylmercury; differentiation of free and bound methylmercuries in biological materials determined by volatility of methylmercury." *Chem Pharm Bull* 1990; 38(5):1412–1413.

Nishiyama, S, et al. "Zinc supplementation alters thyroid hormone metabolism in disabled patients with zinc deficiency." *Jour Amer Coll Nutr* 1994; 13:62–67.

Pansini, F. "Effect of the hormonal contraception on serum reverse triiodothyronine levels." *Gynecol Obstet Invest* 1987; 23:133.

Rachman, B. "Managing endocrine imbalance; autoimmune-induced thyroidopathy and chronic fatigue syndrome." *Functional Medicine Approaches to Endocrine Disturbances of Aging.* Gig Harbor, WA: The Institute for Functional Medicine, 2001.

Rouzier, N. "Estrogen and progesterone replacement." *Longevity and Preventive Medicine Symposium* 2002; 3–8.

Rouzier, N. "Thyroid replacement therapy." *Longevity and Preventive Medicine Symposium* 2002; 16.

Starr, M. *Hypothyroidism Type 2: The Epidemic.* Irvine, CA: New Voice Publications, 2010.

Vliet, E. *Women Weight and Hormones.* New York: Evans & Co, 2001.

Vunevicius, R, et al. "Effects of thyroxine as compared with thyroxine plus triiodothyroxine in patients with hypothyroidism." *NEJM* 1999; 340:424–429.

Woeber, K. "Levothyroxine therapy and serum free thyroxine and free triiodothyronine concentrations." *Jour Endocrinol Invest* 2002; 25(2):106–109.

Chapter 11. Toxic Buildup

Genova Diagnostic Laboratory. www.genovadiagnostics.com

Hanaway, P. "Optimizing Gut Function." *Module III, Fellowship in Anti-Aging and Functional Medicine,* 2006.

Lazarou, J, et al. "Incidence of adverse drug reaction in hospitalized patients." *JAMA* 1998; 279(15):1200–1205.

Sahley, B. *Heal with Amino Acids and Nutrients.* San Antonio: Pain & Stress Publications, 2000.

Vom Saal, F, et al. "Chapel Hill bisphenol A expert panel consensus statement: Integration of mechanisms effects in animals and potential to impact human health at current levels of exposure." *Reprod Toxicol* 2007; 24:131–138.

Chapter 12. Yeast Infection

Agarwal, K. "Therapeutic actions of garlic constitutents." *Med Res Rev* 1996; 16(1):111–124.

Appleton, N. *Stopping Inflammation: Relieving the Cause of Degenerative Diseases.* Garden City Park, NY: Square One Publishers, 2005.

Aziz, N, et al. "Comparative antibacterial and antifungal effects of some phenolic compounds." *Microbios* 1998; 93:43–54.

Blumental, M, Ed. *The Complete German Commission E Monographs: Therapeutic Guide to Herbal Medicines.* Boston: American Botanical Council, 1995.

Crook, W. *The Yeast Connection Handbook.* Jackson, TN: Professional Books, Inc., 2002.

Gruenwald, J, et al. *PDR for Herbal Medicine,* First Edition. Montvale, NJ: Medical Economics Company, 1998.

McLain, N, et al. "Undecylenic acid inhibits morphogenesis of *Candida albicans.*" *Antimicrob Agents Chemother* 2000; 44:2873—2875.

Pieroni, A, et al. "In vitro anti-complementary activity of flavonoids from olive (*Olea europaea L.*) leaves." *Pharmazie* 1996; 51:765–768.

Ponikau, J, et al. "The diagnosis and incidence of allergic fungal sinusitis." *Mayo Clinic Proceedings* 1999; 74:877–884.

Chapter 13. Depression and Antidepressants

Birdsall, T, et al. "5-hydroxytrytophan: a clinically-effective serotonin precursor." *Alter Med Rev* 1998; 3(4):271–280.

Bottiglieri, T, et al. "Folate, vitamin B_{12}, and neuropsychiatric disorders." *Nut Rev* 1996; 54(12):383–390.

Copper, A, et al. "Enhancement of the antidepressant action of fluoxetine by folic acid: a randomized placebo controlled trial." *J Affective Dis* 2000; 60:121–130.

Crayhon, R. *Designs for Health Institute's Eating and Supplement Plans.* Boulder, CO: Designs for Health Institute, 2000.

Edwards, R, et al. "Omega-3 polyunsaturated fatty acids levels in the diet and RBC membranes of depressed patients." *J Affective Dis* 1998; 48:149–155.

Ernst, E, et al. "Adverse effects profile of the herbal antidepressant St. John's wort (*Hypercium perforatum L*)." *Eur J Clin Pharmacol* 1998; 54:589–594.

Galland, L. "Neuroendocrine imbalance in patient care." *Functional Medicine Approaches to Endocrine Disturbances of Aging.* Gig Harbor, WA: The Institute for Functional Medicine, 2001.

Garzya, G, et al. "Evaluation of the effects of L-acetyl carnitine on senile patients suffering from depression." *Drugs Exp Clin Res* 1990; 16:101–106.

Hays, B. "Estrogen and depression." *Disorders of the Brain: Emerging Therapies in Complex Neurologic and Psychiatric Conditions.* Gig Harbor, WA: The Institute for Functional Medicine, 2002.

Hedaya, R. *The Antidepressant Survival Guide.* New York: Three Rivers Press, 2000.

Linde, K, et al. "St John's wort for depression—an overview and meta-analysis of randomized clinical trials." *Br Med J* 1996; 313:253–258.

Maes, M, et al. "Lowered omega-3 polyunsaturated fatty acids in serum phospholipids and cholestreyl esters of depressed patients." *Psychiatry Res* 1999; 85:275–291.

Mehta, A, et al. "Pharmacologic effects of Withania somnifera root extract on GABA receptor complex." *Indian J Med Res* 1991; 94:213–215.

Penninx, B, et al. "Vitamin B_{12} deficiency and depression in physically disabled older women: epidemiological evidence from the women's health and aging study." *Am J Psy* 2000; 157:715–721.

Sahley, B. *Anxiety Epidemic.* San Antonio: Pain & Stress Publications, 1999.

Sakina, M, et al. "A psycho-neuropharmacological profile of centella asiatica extract." *Fitoterrpin* 1990; LXI(4):291–296.

Tempesta, E, et al. "L-acetylcarnitine in depressed elderly subjects. A cross-over study vs. placebo." *Drugs Exp Clin Res* 1987; 13:417–423.

Werbach, M. *Nutritional Influences on Mental Illness: A Sourcebook of Clinical Research.* Tarzana, CA: Third Line Press, Inc, 1991.

Chapter 14. Female Hormone Imbalance

Ahene, S, et al. "Polycystic ovary syndrome." *Nurs Stand* 2004; 18(26):40–44.

Aldercreatz, J, et al. "Western diet and western diseases: some hormonal and biochemical mechanisms and associations." *Scand Jour Clin Lab Invest* 1990; 50 (Suppl 201).

Anderson, B, et al. "Estrogen replacement therapy decreases hyperandrogenicity and improves glucose homeostasis: Plasma lipids in postmenopausal women with NIDDM." *Jour Clin Endocrin* 1997; 82(2):638–643.

Arnot, B. *The Breast Cancer Prevention Diet.* New York: Little Brown and Co, 1998.

Atimo, W, et al. "Familial associations in women with polycystic ovary syndrome." *Fert Steril* 2003; 80(1):143–145.

Baghurst, P, et al. "Diet, prolactin and breast cancer." *Amer Jour Clin Nutr* 1992; 56:943–949.

Barnea, E, et al. "Stress-related reproductive failure." *Jour IVF Embryo Transfer* 1991; 8:15–23.

Bland, J. "Introduction to neuroendocrine disorders." *Functional Medicine Approaches to Endocrine Disturbances of Aging.* Gig Harbor, WA: The Institute for Functional Medicine, 2001.

Bradlow, H, et al. "Effects of pesticides on the ratio of 16-alpha: 2-hydroxyestrone: a biologic marker of breast cancer risk." *Environ Health Prospect* 1995; 103(Suppl 17):147–150.

Bradlow, H, et al. "2-hydroxyestrone the 'good' estrogen." *Jour Endocrinol* 1996; 150 (Suppl): S259–S265.

Brincat, M, et al. "Sex hormones and skin collagen content in postmenopausal woman." *Brit Med Jour* 1983; 287(6402):1337–1338.

Brownstein, D. *Overcoming Thyroid Disorders.* West Bloomfield, MI: Medical Alternatives Press, 2002.

Carey, A, et al. "Evidence for a single gene effect causing polycystic ovaries and male pattern baldness." *Clin Endocrinol* 38(6):653–658.

Clarkson, T, et al. "Conjugated equine estrogens alone, but not in combination with medroxyprogesterone acetate, inhibit aortic connective tissue remodeling after plasma lipid lowering in female monkeys." *Arterioscler Thromb Vasc Biol* 1998; 18(7):1164–1171.

Colacurci, N, et al. "Effects of hormone replacement therapy on glucose metabolism." *Panminerva Med* 1998; 40(1):18–21.

Colditz, G, et al. "Use of estrogen plus progestin is associated with greater increase in breast cancer risk than estrogen alone." *Amer Jour Epidemiol* 1998; 147(Suppl):64S.

Collins, J. *What's Your Menopause Type?* Roseville, CA: Prima Health, 2000.

Davis, S, et al. "Use of androgens in postmenopausal women." *Curr Opin Obstet Gynecol* 1997; 9(3):177–180.

De Leo, V, et al. "Polycystic ovary syndrome and type 2 diabetes mellitus." *Minera Ginecol* 2004; 56(1):53–62.

"Drugs that cause sexual dysfunction: an update." *The Medical Letter* 1992; 34 (Issue 876).

Ellison, P, et al. "Measurements of salivary progesterone." *Ann of the New York Acad of Sci* 1993; 694:161–176.

Falola, E, et al. "Body composition, fat distribution and metabolic characteristics in lean and obese women with polycystic ovary syndrome." *Jour Endocrinol Invest* 2004; 27(5):424–429.

Fishman, J, et al. "Biological properties of 16-alpha hydroxyl estrone: implications in estrogen physiology and pathophysiology." *Jour Clin Endocrinol Metabol* 1980; 51:611–615.

Fishman, J, et al. "Increased estrogen 16-alpha hydroxylase activity in women with breast and endometrial cancer." *Jour Steroid Biochem* 1984; 20:1077–1081.

Fishman, J, et al. "The role of estrogen in mammary carcinogenesis." *Ann NY Acad Sci* 1995; 768:63, 91–100.

Follingstad, A. "Estriol, the forgotten estrogen?" *JAMA* 1978; 239(1):29–30.

Gambineria, A, et al. "Obesity and the polycystic ovary syndrome." *Int Jour Obes Relat Metab Disord* 2002; 26(7):883–896.

Gerhard, M, et al. "Estradiol therapy combined wit progesteterone; endothelium-dependent vasodilation in postmenopausal women." *Circulation* 1998; 98(12):1158–1163.

Gonzalez, C, et al. "Polycystic ovarian disease: clinical and biochemical expression." *Ginecol Obstet Mex* 2003; 71:253–258.

Gonzalez, C, et al. "Polycystic ovaries in childhood: a common finding in daughters of PCOS patients. A pilot study." *Hum Repro* 2002; 17(3):771–776.

Haffner, S, et al. "Endogenous sex hormones: impact on lipids, lipoproteins, and insulin." *Amer Jour Med* 1995; 98(1A):40S–47S.

Harris, C, and T Cheung. *The PCOS Protection Plan.* Carlsbad, CA: Hay House, Inc, 2006.

Henderson, B, et al. "Estrogen replacement therapy and protection from acute MI." *Amer Jour Obstet Gynecol* 1988; 159:312–317.

Hofman, T, et al. "Steroid hormones in saliva." *Diagnostic Endocrinol Met* 1998; 16(9):265–273.

Kalkoff, R, et al. "Metabolic effects of progesterone." *Jour Obstect Gynecol* 1982; 142–146, 735–738.

Khaw, K, et al. "Fasting plasma glucose levels and endogenous androgens in non-diabetic postmenopausal women." *Clin Sci* 1991; 80(3):199–203.

Laux, M. *Natural Woman, Natural Menopause.* New York: HarperCollins, 1997.

Lee, J. *What Your Doctor May Not Tell You About Menopause.* New York: Warner Books, 1996.

Lee, J. *What Your Doctor May Not Tell You About Premenopause.* New York: Warner Books, 1999.

Legro, R, et al. "Prevalence and predictors of risk for Type 2 diabetes mellitus and impaired glucose tolerance in polycystic ovary syndrome: a prospective, controlled study in 254 affected women." *Jour Clin Endocrinol Metabol* 1999; 84(1):165–169.

Lemon, H, et al. "Estriol prevention of mammary carcinoma induced by 7, 12–dimethylbenzanthracene and procarbazine." *Cancer Res* 1975; 35:1341–1352.

Lemon, H, et al. "Pathophysiologic considerations in the treatment of menopausal symptoms with estrogens: the role of estriol in the prevention of mammary carcinoma." *ACTA Endocrinol* 1980; 233 (Suppl):17–27.

Lemon, H, et al. "Reduced estriol excretion in patients with breast cancer prior to endocrine therapy." *JAMA* 1966; 196(13):1129–1136.

Luck, M, et al. "Ascorbic acid and fertility." *Biol Reproduc* 1995; 52:262–265.

Majewska, M, et al. "Steroid hormone metabolites are barbiturate-like modulators of the GABA receptor." *Science* 1986; 232:1004.

Mandel, I, et al. "The diagnostic use of saliva." *Jour Oral Pathol Med* 1990; 19:119–125.

Manvais-Jarvis, P, et al. "Progesterone and progestins: a general overview." *Progesterone and Progestins*. New York: Rave Press, 1983.

Marantides, D, et al. "Management of polycystic ovary syndrome." *Nurse Pract* 1997; 22(12):34–38, 40–41.

Martucci, C, et al. "P450 enzymes of estrogen metabolism." *Pharmacol Ther* 1993; 57:237–257.

Meilahn, D. "Do urinary oestrogen metabolites predict breast cancer?" *Guersey III Cohort Follow-up* 1998; 78(9):1250–1255.

Melton, L, et al. "Progestins reverse some of the effects of estrogen." *TEM* 2000; 11(2):69–71.

Michnovicz, J, et al. "Introduction of estradiol metabolism by dietary indole-3-carbinol in humans." *Jour Nat Canc Inst* 1990; 82:947–949.

Minshall, R, et al. "Ovarian steroid protection against coronary artery hyperreactivity in rhesus monkeys." *Jour Clin Endocrinol Metab* 1998; 83(2):649–659.

Miodrg, A, et al. "Sex hormones and the female urinary tract." *Drugs* 1988; 36(4):491–504.

Murray, M. *The Healing Power of Herbs*. Roseville, CA: Prima Publications, 1995.

Nutrition and Healing Newsletter, 1995; Vol. 11, No.12.

Ottoson, U, et al. "Oral progesterone and estrogen/progestogen therapy; effects of natural and synthetic hormones on subfractions of HDL cholesterol and liver proteins." *ACTA Obstet Cynecol Scand* 1984; (Suppl), 127:1–37.

Ottoson, U, et al. "Subfractions of high-density lipo-protein cholesterol during estrogen replacement therapy: A comparison between progestogens and natural progesterone." *Jour of Obstetrics and Gynec* 1985; 151:746–750.

Pansini, F, et al. "Control of carbohydrate metabolism in menopausal women receiving transdermal estrogen therapy." *Ann NY Acad Sci* 1990; 592:460–462.

Panth, M, et al. "Effect of vitamin A supplementation on plasma progesterone and estradiol levels during pregnancy." *Int Jour Vit Nutr Res* 1991; 61.

Pelusi, B, et al. "Type 2 diabetes and the polycystic ovary syndrome." *Minerva Ginecol* 2004; 56(1):41–51.

Persky, H. "Plasma testosterone level and sexual behavior of couples." *Arch Sex Behav* 1978; 7(3):157–73.

The Postmenopausal Estrogen/Progestin Interventions (PEPI) trial: National Heart, Lung, and Blood Institute, Nov. 17, 1994; 1–4.

Prior, J, et al. "Progesterone as a bone-tropic hormone." *Endocrine Reviews* 1990; 11:386–398.

Riad-Fahney, L, et al. "Steroids in saliva for assessing endocrine function." *Endocrine Reviews* 1982; 3(4):367–395.

Robinson, S, et al. "Postprandial thermogenesis is reduced in polycystic ovary syndrome and is associated with increased insulin resistance." *Clin Endocrinol* (Oxf) 1992; 36(6):537–543.

Ross, R, et al. "Effect of hormone replacement therapy on breast cancer risk: estrogen versus estrogen plus progestin." *Jour Natl Cancer Inst* 1992; (4):328–332.

Rouzier, N. "Estrogen and progesterone replacement." *Longevity and Preventive Medicine Symposium* 2002; 12–14.

Sacks, F, et al. "Sex hormones, lipoproteins, and vascular reactivity." *Curr Opin Lipodol* 1995; 6(3):161–166.

Sand, R, et al. "Exogenous androgens in postmenopausal women." *Amer Jour of Med* 1995; 98(1A).

Schairer, C, et al. "Menopausal estrogen and estrogen-progestin replacement therapy and breast cancer risk." *JAMA* 2000; 283:485–491.

Schedlowski, M, et al. "Acute psychological stress increases plasma levels of cortisol, prolactin and thyroid stimulating hormone." *Life Sciences* 1992; 50:1201–1205.

Schmidt, J, et al. "Other anti-androgens." *Dermatology* 1998; 196(1):153–157.

Shippen, E. *Testosterone Syndrome.* New York: M. Evans & Company, Inc, 1998.

Sinatra, S. *Heart Sense for Women.* Washington DC: LifeLine Press, 2000.

Smith, P. *HRT: The Answers.* Traverse City, MI: Healthy Living Books, 2003.

Smith, P. *Vitamins: Hype or Hope?* Traverse City, MI: Healthy Living Books, 2004.

Smith, P. *What You Must Know About Women's Hormones.* Garden City Park, NY: Square One Publishers, 2010.

Solomon, C, et al. "Long or irregular menstrual cycle as a marker for the risk of type 2 diabetes mellitus." *JAMA* 2001; 286(19):2421–2426.

Stefanick, M, et al. "Estrogen, progestogens and cardiovascular risk: review of PEPPI trial." *Jour Repro Med* 1999; 44(Suppl):221–226.

Strauss, J, et al. "Some new thoughts on the pathophysiology and genetics of polycystic ovary syndrome." *Ann NY Aci Sci* 2003; 997:42–48.

Surrel, P, et al. "Cardiovascular aspects of androgens in women." *Semin Repro Endocrin* 1998; 16(2):121–128.

Telang, N, et al. "Induction by estrogen metabolite 16-alpha hydroxyl estrone of genotoxic damage and aberrant proliferation in mouse mammary epithelial cells." *Jour Nat Cancer Inst* 1992; 84(8):634–638.

Testosterone: Action, Deficiency, Substitution. Cambridge, UK: Cambridge University Press, 2004.

Tsilchorozidou, T, et al. "Altered cortisol metabolism in polycystic ovary syndrome: insulin enhances 5 alpha-reduction but not the elevated adrenal steroid production rates." *Jour Clin Endocrino Metab* 2003; 88(12):5907–5913.

Urbanek, M, et al. "Thirty-seven candidate genes for PCOS: Strongest evidence of linkage is follistatin." *Proc Nat Acd Aci* 1999; 38(6):653–658.

Ursin, G, et al. "Urinary 2-hydroxy estrone/16 alpha hydroxyl estrone ratio: risk of breast cancer in postmenopausal women." *Jour Nat Canc Inst* 1999; 91:1067–1072.

Vining, R, et al. "Hormones in saliva: mode of entry and consequent implications for clinical interpretation." *Clin Chemistry* 1983; 29(10):1752–1756.

Vining, R, et al. "The measurements of hormones in saliva: possibility and pitfalls." *Jour of Steroid Biochem* 1987; 27:81–94.

Vliet, E. *Women, Weight and Hormones.* New York: M. Evans & Company, 2001.

Zhu, B, et al. "Is 2-methoxyestradiol an endogenous estrogen metabolite that inhibits mammary carcinogenesis?" *Cancer Res* 1998; 58:2269–2277.

Chapter 15. Genes

Bachmanov, A, et al. "Genetics of sweet taste preferences." *Pure Appl Chem* 2002; 74:1135–1140.

Bartoshuk, L. "Comparing sensory experiences across individuals: recent psychophysical advances illuminate genetic variation in taste perception." *Chem Senses* 2000; 25:447–460.

Boughter, J, et al. "Behavioral genetics and taste." *BMC Neurosci* 2007; 8(Suppl 3):S3.

Castle, D, Ed. *Nutrition and Genomics.* New York: Elsevier, 2009.

Chale-Rush, A, et al. "Evidence for human orosensory (taste?) sensitivity to fatty acids." *Chem Senses* 2007; 32:423–431.

Chandrashekar, J, et al. "T2Rs function as bitter taste receptors." *Cell* 2000; 100:703–711.

Chandrashekar, J, et al. "The receptors and cells for mammalian taste." *Nature* 2006; 44:288–294.

Chaudhari, N, et al. "A metabotropic glutamate receptor variant functions as a taste receptor." *Nat Neurosci* 2000; 3:113–119.

Desimone, J, et al. "Taste receptors in the gastrointestinal tract III. Salty and sour taste: sensing of sodium and protons by the tongue." *Am J Physiol Gastrointest Liver Physiol* 2006; 291: G1005–G1010.

Drayna, D. "Human taste genetics." *Annu Rev Genomics Hum Genet* 2005; 6:217–235.

Drewnowski, A, et al. "Genetic taste markers and food preference." *Drug Metabl Dispos* 2001; 29:535–538.

Drewnowski, A, et al. "Taste and food preferences as predictors of dietary practices in young women." *Public Health Nutr* 1999; 2:513—519.

Duffy, V, et al. "Food acceptance and genetic variation in taste." *Jour Amer Diet Assoc* 2000; 100:647–655.

Eisenstein, M. "Taste: more than meets the mouth." *Nature* 2010; 468:S18–S19.

Eny, K, et al. "Genetic variant in the glucose transporter type 2 (GLUT2) is associated with higher intakes of sugars in two distinct populations." *Physiol Genomics* 2008; 33:355—360.

Fushan, A, et al. "Allelic polymorphism within the TAS1R3 promoter is associated with human taste sensitivity to sucrose." *Current Biology* 2009; 19:1268–1293.

Garcia-Bailo, B, et al. "Genetic variation in taste and its influence on food selection." *A Jour of Integrative Biology* 2009; 13(1):69–80.

Heck, G, et al. "Salt taste transduction occurs through an amiloride-sensitive sodium transport pathway." *Science* 1984; 223:403—405.

Horowitz, S. "Nutrigenomics and nutrigenetics: personalized nutrition based on your genes." *Alernat Complement Therapy* 2005; 115–119.

Huang, A, et al. "The cells and logic for mammalian sour taste detection." *Nature* 2006; 442:934–938.

Keskitalo, K, et al. "Same genetic components underlie different measures of sweet taste preference." *Amer Jour Clin Nutr* 2007; 86:1663–1669.

Keskitalo, K, et al. "Sweet taste preferences are partly genetically determined: identification of a trait locus on chromosome." *Amer Jour Clin Nutr* 2007; 86:55–63.

Kim, U, et al. "Genetics of human taste perception." *Jour Dent Res* 2004; 83:448–453.

Kitagawa, M, et al. "Molecular genetic identification of a candidate receptor gene for sweet taste." *Biochem Biophys Res Commun* 2001; 283:236–242.

Kurihara, K, et al. "Physiologic studies on umami taste." *Jour Nutr* 2000; 130:931S–934S.

Laugerette, F, et al. "Do we taste fat?" *Biochimie* 2007; 89:265–269.

Li, X, et al. "Human receptors for sweet and umami taste." *Proc Natl Acad Sci USA* 2002; 99:4692–4696.

Liao, J, et al. "Three sweet receptor genes are clustered in human chromosome 1." *Mamm Genome* 2003; 14:291–301.

Lindemann, B, et al. "The discovery of umami." *Chem Senses* 2002; 27:843–844.

Mela, D, et al. "Sensory preferences for fats: relationships with diet and body composition." *Amer Jour Cln Nutr* 1991; 53:908–915.

Mennella, J, et al. "Genetic and environmental determinants of bitter perception and sweet preferences." *Paediatrics* 2005; 115:216–222.

Nie, Y, et al. "Distinct contributions of T1R2 and T1R3 taste receptor subunits to the detection of sweet stimuli." *Curr Biol* 2005; 15:1948–1951.

Sainz, E, et al. "Identification of a novel member of the T1R family of putative taste receptors." *Jour Neurochem* 2001; 77:896–903.

Ugawa, S, et al. "Receptor that leaves a sour taste in the mouth." *Nature* 1998; 395:555–556.

Chapter 16. Insulin Resistance

Ali, L., et al. "Characterization of the hypoglycemic effects of *Trigonella foenum graecum* seed." *Planta Med* 1995; 61:358–360.

Anderson, R, et al. "Chromium, glucose tolerance, and diabetes." *Jour Amer Coll Nutr* 1998; 17(6):548–55.

Baskaran, K, et al. "Antidiabetic effect of a leaf extract form Gymnema sylvestre in non-insulin-dependent diabetes mellitus patients." *Jour Ethnopharmacol* 1990; 30:295–305.

Berrio, L, et al. "Insulin activity: stimulatory effects of cinnamon and Brewer's yeast as influenced by albumin." *Horm Res* 1992; 37:225–229.

Brewerton, T, et al. "Toward a unified theory of serotonin dysregulation in eating and related disorders." *Psychoneuroendocrin* 1995; 20: 561–590.

Elder, C. "Ayurveda for diabetes mellitus: a review of the biomedical literature." *Alternative Therapies* 2004; 10(1):44–50.

Facchini, F, et al. "Insulin resistance and cigarette smoking." *Lancet* 1992; 339:1128—1130.

Foster-Powell, K, et al. "International tables of glycemic index." *Amer Jour of Clin Nutrition* 1995; 62:871S–893S.

Friedman, T, et al. "Carbohydrate and lipid metabolism in endogenous hypercortisolism: shared features with metabolic syndrome X and NIDDM." *Endocr Jour* 1996; 43:645–655.

Houston, M. "The metabolic syndrome: pathophysiology, diagnosis, clinical aspects, prevention and nonpharmacologic treatment: emphasis on lifestyle modifications, nutrition, nutritional supplements, vitamins, minerals, antioxidants, weight management and exercise." *JANA* 2005; 8(2):7.

Kaczmar, T. "Herbal support for diabetes management." *Clinical Nutrition Insights* 1998; 6(8):1–4.

Khan, A, et al. "Insulin potentiating factor and chromium content of selected foods and spices." *Biol Trace Element Res* 1990; 24:183–188.

Madar, Z, et al. "Glucose-lowering effect of fenugreek in non-insulin dependent diabetics." *Eur Jour Clin Nutr* 1988; 42:51–54.

Marles, F, et al. "Antidiabetic plants and their active constituents: an update." *Protocol Jour Nat Med* 1996; 85:111.

Mertz, W, et al. "Interaction of chromium with insulin: a progress report." *Nutr Rev* 1998; 56:174–177.

Meyer, K, et al. "Carbohydrates, dietary fiber and incidence of type II diabetes in older women." *Amer Jour Clin Nutr* 2000; 71:921–930.

Nilsson, P, et al. "Adverse effects of psychosocial stress on gonadal function and insulin levels in middle-aged males." *Jour Inter Med* 1995; 237:479–486.

Pereira M, et al. *JAMA* 2004; 292(20):2482–2490.

Raikkonen, K, et al. "Psychosocial stress and the insulin resistance syndrome." *Metabolism* 1996; 45:1533–1538.

Salmeron, J, et al. "Dietary fiber, glycemic load, and risk of non-insulin dependent diabetes mellitus in women." *JAMA* 1997; 277:472–477.

Schwarzbein, D. *The Schwarzbein Principle II*. Deerfield Beach, FL: Health Communications, 2002.

Sharma, R, et al. "Effect of fenugreek seeds on blood glucose and serum insulin responses in human subjects." *Nutr Res* 1986; 6:1353–1364.

Smith, P. *Vitamins: Hype or Hope*. Traverse City, MI: Healthy Living Books, 2004.

Stivastava, Y, et al. "Antidiabetic and adaptogenic properties of *Momordica charantia* extract: an experimental and clinical evaluation." *Phytotherapy Res* 1993; 7:285–289.

Targher, G, et al. "Cigarette smoking and insulin resistance in patients with non-insulin dependent diabetes mellitus." *Jour of Endocrinology and Metabol* 1997; 82:3619–3624.

Vitelli, L, et al. "Association of dietary composition with fasting serum insulin level: the ARIC Study." *Nutr Metab Cardiovasc Disc* 1996; 81:892–997.

Vliet, E. *Women, Weight and Hormones*. New York: Evans & Company, 2001.

Yeh, G, et al. "Systemic review of herbs and dietary supplements for glycemic control in diabetes." *Diabetic Care* 2003; 26(4):1277–1294.

Chapter 17. Male Hormone Deficiency

Alexander, G, et al. "Androgen-behavior correlations in hypogonadal men and eugonadal men. II. Cognitive abilities." *Hormones and Behavior* 1998; 33(2):85–94.

Baran, D, et al. "Effect of testosterone therapy on bone formation in an osteoporotic hypogonadal male." *Calcified Tissue Res* 1978; 26:103–106.

Barrett-Connor, E, et al. "Endogenous sex hormones and cognitive function in older men." *Jour Clin Endocrin Metabol* 1999; 84(10):3681–3685.

Bhasin, S. "The dose-dependent effects of testosterone on sexual function and on muscle mass and function." *Mayo Clin Proc* 2000; Jan. 75 (Suppl: S70–S75).

Boyanov, M, et al. "Testosterone supplementation in men with type 2 diabetes, visceral obesity and partial androgen deficiency." *Aging Male* 2003; 6(1):1–7.

Burris, A, et al. "A long-term prospective study of the physiology and behavioral effects of hormone replacement in untreated hypogonadal men." *Jour Androl* 1992; 13(4):297–304.

Channer, K, et al. "Cardiovascular effects of testosterone: implications of the 'male menopause'?" *Heart* 2003; 89(2):121–122.

Gouras, G, et al. "Testosterone reduces neuronal secretion of Alzheimer's beta-amyloid peptides." *Proc Nat Acad Sci USA* 97(3):1202–1205.

Hak, A, et al. "Low levels of endogenous androgens increase the risk of atherosclerosis in elderly men: The Rotterdam Study." *Jour of Clin Endocrin & Metabol* 2002; 87(8):3632–3639.

Hogervorst, E, et al. "Low free testosterone is an independent risk factor for Alzheimer's disease." *Exp Gerontol* 2004; 39(11–12):1633–1639.

Jackson, J, et al. "Testosterone deficiency as a risk factor for hip fractures in men: a case-control study." *Amer Jour of Med Sci* 1992; 304:4–8.

Korenman, S, et al. "Secondary hypogonadism in older men: Its relationship to impotence." *Jour Clin Endocrin Metab* 1990; 71:963–969.

Malkin, C, et al. "The effect of testosterone replacement on endogenous inflammatory cytokines and lipid profiles in hypogonadal men." *Jour Clin Endocrinology Metab* 2004; 89(7):3313–3318.

Malkin, C, et al. "Testosterone as a protective factor against atherosclerosis—immunomodulation and influence upon plaque development and stability." *Jour Endocrinolo* 2003; 78(3):373–380.

Moffat, S, et al. "Long-term measures of free testosterone predict regional cerebral blood flow patterns in elderly men." *Neurobiol Aging* 2006; May 11.

Muller, M, et al. "Endogenous sex hormones and progression of carotid atherosclerosis in elderly men." *Circulation* 2004; 109(17):2074–2079.

Murphy, S, et al. "Sex hormones and bone mineral density in elderly men." *Bone Mineral* 1993; 20:133–140.

Rothenberg, R. "Testosterone Replacement Therapy: Male Menopause." *Fellowship in Anti-Aging and Functional Medicine: Module I.* Las Vegas, December 2006.

Shippen, E. *The Testosterone Syndrome.* New York: M. Evans and Company, 1998.

Tan, R. "A pilot study on the effects of testosterone in hypogonadal aging male patients with Alzheimer's disease." *Aging Male* 2003; 6(1):13–17.

Webb, C, et al. "Effects of testosterone on coronary vasomotor regulation in men with coronary heart disease." *Circulation* 1999; 100(16):1690–1696.

Chapter 18. Neurotransmitter Dysfunction

Birdsall, T. "5–hydroxytryptophan: A clinically-effective serotonin precursor." *Alt Med Rev* 1998; 3:271–278.

Birdsall, T. "Therapeutic applications of taurine." *Altern Med Rev* 1998; 3:128–136.

Blaylock, R. *Excitotoxins: The Taste That Kills.* Santa Fe: Health Press, 1997.

Bond, A, et al. "Tryptophan depletion increases aggression in women during the premenstrual phase." *Psychopharm* (Berl) 2001; 156(4):477–480.

Chapman, R, et al. "Taurine and the heart." *Cardiovasc Res* 1993; 27(3):358–363.

Collins, B. "Plasma and urinary taurine in epilepsy." *Clin Chem* 1988; 34(4):671–675.

Crayhon, R. "Aging well in the 21st century." *Seminar* 2002.

Dawson, R. "An age-related decline in striatal taurine is correlated with a loss of dopaminergic markers." *Brain Res Bull* 199; 48:319–324.

Delgado, P, et al. "Role of norepinephrine in depression." *Jour Clin Psychiatry* 2000; 61:(Suppl 1):5–12.

den Boer, J, et al. "Behavior, neuroendocrine, and biochemical effects of 5-hydroxytryptophan administration in panic disorder." *Psychiatry Res* 1990; 31:267–278.

Desai, T, et al. "Taurine deficiency after intensive chemotherapy and/or radiation." *Amer Jour Clin Nutr* 1992; 55(3):708–711.

Efron, D, et al. "Role of arginine in immunonutrition." *Jour Gastroenterol* 2000; 35(suppl 12):20–23.

Fujita, T, et al. "Hypotensive effect of taurine, possible involvement of the sympathetic nervous system and endogenous opiates." *Jour Clin Invest* 1988; 82(3):993–997.

Gaby, A. *Nutritional Therapy in Medical Practice.* Carlisle, PA: Nutrition Seminars, 2003.

Hamon, M, et al. "Role of serotonin and other neuroactive molecules in the physiopathogenesis of migraine." *Pathol Bio* (Paris) 2000; 48(7):619–629.

Huxtable, R, et al. "Physiologic actions of taurine." *Physiol Rev* 1992; 72:101–163.

Keast, D, et al. "Depression of plasma glutamine concentration after exercise stress and its possible influence on the immune system." *Med Jour Aust* 1995; 162(1):15–18.

Kendler, B, et al. "Taurine: an overview of its role in preventive medicine." *Prev Med* 1989; 18(1):70–100.

Klatz, R. *The New Anti-Aging Revolution*. North Bergen, NJ: Basic Health Publications, 2003.

Kumata, K, et al. "Restoration of endothelium-dependent relaxation in both hypercholesterolemic and diabetics by chronic taurine." *Eur Jour Pharmacol* 1996; 303:47–53.

LeDoux, J. *Synaptic Self: Our Brains Become Who We Are*. New York: Penguin Books, 2002.

Lee, Z, et al. "Urinary epinephrine and norepinephrine interrelations with obesity, insulin, and the metabolic syndrome in Hong Kong Chinese." *Metabolism* 2001; 50(2):135–143.

Lombardini, J, et al. "Taurine retinal function." *Brain Res Rev* 1991; 16(2):151–169.

Maskovitz, B, et al. "Glutamine metabolism and utilization: relevance to major problems in health care." *Pharmacol Res* 1994; 30(1):61–71.

Meguid, M, et al. "Hypothalamic dopamine and serotonin in the regulation of food intake." *Nutrition* 2000; 16(10):843–857.

Nakagawa, M, et al. "Antihypertensive effect of taurine on the salt-induced hypertension." *Adv Exp Med Biol* 1994; 359:197–206.

Nester, E. *Molecular NeuroPharmacology*. New York: McGraw-Hill, 2001.

Nurjhan, N, et al. "Glutamine: a major gluconeogenic precursor and vehicle for interorgan carbon transport in man." *Jour Clin Invest* 1995; 95(1):272–277.

Peck, L, et al. "Glutamine should be figured into inflammatory bowel disease formulations." *Family Practice News* June 1994.

Redmond, H, et al. "Immunonutrition: the role of taurine." *Nutrition* 1998; 14(7–8):599–604.

Ribeiro, C, et al. "5-hydroxytryptophan in the prophylaxis of chronic tension-type headache: a double-blind, random, placebo-controlled study for the Portuguese Head Society." *Headache* 2000; 40:451–456.

Rosenbaum, M, et al. "Effects of changes in body weight on carbohydrate metabolism, catecholamine excretion, and thyroid function." *Amer Jour Clin Nutr* 2000; 71(6):1421–1432.

Sahley, B. *The Anxiety Amino Acid*. San Antonio: Pain & Stress Publications, 1999.

Sahley, B. *Healing with Amino Acids and Nutrients*. San Antonio: Pain & Stress Publications, 2000.

Shabert, J, et al. *The Ultimate Nutrient Glutamine*. Garden City Park, NY: Avery Publishing Group, 1994.

Siani, A, et al. "Blood pressure and metabolic changes during dietary L-arginine supplementation in humans." *Amer Jour Hypertens* 2000; 13(5, Pt. 1):547–551.

Sinatra, S. *Heart Sense for Women*. Washington, DC: LifeLine Press, 2000.

von Bohlen und Halback, O. *Neurotransmitters and Neuromodultors*. 2002.

Waagepetersen, H, et al. "The GABA paradox: multiple roles as a metabolite, neurotransmitter and neurodifferentiative agent." *Jour Neurochem* 1999; 73(4):1335–1342.

Welbourne, T, et al. "Increased plasma bicarbonate and growth hormone after an oral glutamine load." *Amer Jour Clin Nutr* 1995; 61(5):1058–1061.

Zackheim, H, et al. "Taurine and psoriasis." *Jour Invest Dermatol* 1968; 50(23):277–230.

Chapter 19. Pregnenolone Insufficiency

Ravnskov, U. *The Cholesterol Myths*. Winona, Lake, IN: New Trends Publishing, 2000.

Roberts, E, et al. "Pregnenolone—from Selye to Alzheimer's and a model of the pregnenolone sulfate finding site on the GABAA receptor." *Biochemical Pharm* 1995; 49(1):1–16.

Sahelian, R. *Pregnenolone: Nature's Feel Good Hormone*. Garden City Park, NY: Avery Publishing, 1997.

Yanick, P. *Prohormone Nutrition*. Montclair, NJ: Longevity Institute International, 1998.

Young, D. *Pregnenolone: A Radical New Approach to Health, Longevity, and Emotional Well-Being*. Salem, UT: Essentials Science Publishing, 2000.

Chapter 20. Putting It All Together

Bateman, J, et al. "Possible toxicity of herbal remedies." *Scottish Med Jour* 1998; 4:7–15.

Belury, M, et al. "Conjugated dienoic linoleate: a polyunsaturated fatty acid with unique chemo-protective properties." *Nur Res* 1995; 53(4 Pt. 1):83–89.

Berkey, C, et al. "Milk, dairy fat, dietary calcium, and weight gain: a longitudinal study of adolescents." *Arch Pediatr Adolesc Med* 2005; 159(6):543–550.

Bland, J. *Applying Functional Medicine in Clinical Practice*. Gig Harbor, WA: Institute for Functional Medicine, 2002.

Bland, J. *Clinical Nutrition: A Functional Approach*. Gig Harbor, WA: Institute for Functional Medicine, 1999.

Blankson, H, et al. "Conjugated linoleic acid reduces body fat mass in overweight and obese humans." *Jour Nutr* 2000; 130(12):2943–2948.

Colgan, M. *The New Nutrition*. Vancouver, Canada: Apple Publishing, 1995.

Crayhon, R. *The Carnitine Miracle*. New York: M. Evans and Company, 1998.

Doyle, L, et al. "Scientific forum explores CLA knowledge." *Inform* 1998; 9(1):69.

Epstein, F, et al. "Glucose transporters and insulin action: implication for insulin resistance and diabetes mellitus." *NEJM* 1999; 341(4):248–257.

Fuhr, U, et al. "Drug interactions with grapefruit juice, extent, probable mechanism, and clinical relevance." *Drug Sci* 1998; 18:251—272.

Gaby, A. *Nutritional Therapy in Medical Practice*. Carlisle, PA: Nutrition Seminars, 2003.

Galland. L. "Person-centered diagnosis and chronic fatigue." *Metabolic Energy, Messenger Molecules, and Chronic Illness: The Functional Perspective*. Gig Harbor, WA: Institute for Functional Medicine, 2000.

Hart, C. *The Insulin-Resistance Diet*. Chicago: Contemporary Books, 2001.

Klatz, R. *The New Anti-Aging Revolution*. North Bergen, NJ: Basic Health Publications, 2003.

Lieberman, S. *The Real Vitamin ad Mineral Book*. Garden City Park, NY: Avery Publishing Group, 1997.

Meletis, C. *Interactions Between Drugs and Natural Medicines*. Sandy, OR: Electric Medical Publications, 1999.

Moreira, P, et al. "Dietary calcium and body mass index in Portuguese children." *Eur Jour Clin Nutr* 2005; May 25.

Moya-Camarena, S, et al. "Conjugated linoleic acid is a potent naturally occurring ligand and activator of PPAR." *Jour Lipid Res* 1999; 40:1426–1433.

Murray, C, et al. "Alternative projections of mortality and disability by cause 1990–2020: global burden of disease study." *Lancet* 1997; 349:1498–1504.

Pariza, M, et al. "Conjugated dienoic derivatives of linolic acid: a new class of anticarcinogerns." *Med Oncol Tumor Pharmacother* 1990; 7(2–3):169–171.

Riserus, U, et al. "Conjugated linoleic acid (CLA) reduced abdominal adipose tissue in obese middle-aged men with signs of metabolic syndrome: a randomized controlled trial." *Int Jour Obes Related Metab Disord* 2001; 25(8):1129–1135.

Ryder, J, et al. "Isomer-specific antidiabetic properties of conjugated linoleic acid. Improve glucose tolerance skeletal muscle insulin action, and UCP-2 gene expression." *Diabetes* 2001; 50:1149–1157.

Sahley, B. *Heal with Amino Acids and Nutrients.* San Antonio: Pain & Stress Publications, 2000.

Tanphaichitr, V, et al. "Carnitine metabolism and human carnitine deficiency." *Nutrition* 1993; 9:246–254.

Ulene, A. *Dr. Art Ulene's Complete Guide to Vitamins, Minerals, and Herbs.* Garden City Park, NY: Avery Publishing, 2000.

Young, G. *Ningxia Wolfberry: The Ultimate Superfood.* Orem, UT: Essential Science Publishing, 2006.

Index

A

Acute inflammation, 71. *See also* Chronic inflammation.
Adrenal fatigue, 46–47
Adrenaline. *See* Epinephrine.
Aerobic exercise, 16. *See also* Exercise.
Agmatine, 172
Agricultural grade supplements, 197
Allergen, 66
Allergenic foods. *See* Food allergies.
Amino acids, 7
Amish, genetic makeup of, 149
Anaerobic exercise, 16. *See also* Exercise.
Anaphylaxis, 66
Androgens, 128, 163. *See also* Testosterone.
Andropause, 163
Antibodies and food allergies, 66, 69
Antidepressants, 118–119, 166
Aromatase, 167
Asbestos, 92
Aspartic acid, 173

B

Bariatric surgeons, 203
Biochemical factor questionnaire. *See* Self-tests for determining cause of weight gain.
Biochemical factors affecting weight. *See* Depression; Female hormonal imbalance; Genes; Insulin resistance; Male hormone deficiency; Neurotransmitter dysfunction; Pregnenolone insufficiency.

C

Calories, 10
burned, during various activities, 19
Candida Immune Complex Assay, 107
Candida yeast, different species of, 103
Candidiasis. *See* Yeast infection.
Chefs, personal, 193–194
Chlorine, 92
Chronic depression. *See* Depression.

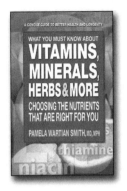
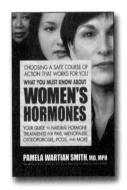

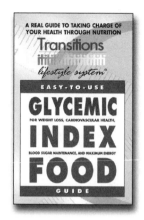

GLYCEMIC INDEX FOOD GUIDE
For Weight Loss, Cardiovascular Health, Diabetic Management, and Maximum Energy
Dr. Shari Lieberman

The glycemic index (GI) is an important nutritional tool. By indicating how quickly a given food triggers a rise in blood sugar, the GI enables you to choose foods that can help you manage a variety of conditions and improve your overall health.

Written by leading nutritionist Dr. Shari Lieberman, this book was designed as an easy-to-use guide to the glycemic index. The book first answers commonly asked questions, ensuring that you truly understand the GI and know how to use it. It then provides both the glycemic index and the glycemic load of hundreds of foods and beverages, including raw foods, cooked foods, and many combination and prepared foods. Whether you are interested in controlling your glucose levels to manage your diabetes, lose weight, increase your heart health, or simply enhance your well-being, the *Glycemic Index Food Guide* is the best place to start.

$7.95 US • 160 pages • 4 x 7-inch mass paperback • ISBN 978-0-7570-0245-8

THE ACID-ALKALINE FOOD GUIDE
A Quick Reference to Foods & Their Effect on pH Levels
Dr. Susan E. Brown and Larry Trivieri, Jr.

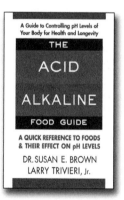

In the last few years, researchers around the world have reported the importance of acid-alkaline balance to good health. While thousands of people are trying to balance their body's pH level, until now, they have had to rely on guides containing only a small number of foods. *The Acid-Alkaline Food Guide* is a complete resource for people who want to widen their food choices.

The book begins by explaining how the acid-alkaline environment of the body is influenced by foods. It then presents a list of thousands of foods—single foods, combination foods, and even fast foods—and their acid-alkaline effects. *The Acid-Alkaline Food Guide* will quickly become the resource you turn to at home, in restaurants, and whenever you want to select a food that can help you reach your health and dietary goals.

$7.95 US • 208 pages • 4 x 7-inch mass paperback • ISBN 978-0-7570-0280-9

A Guide to Complementary Treatments for Diabetes

Using Natural Supplements, Nutrition, and Alternative Therapies to Better Manage Your Diabetes

Gene Bruno, MS, MHS

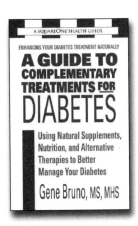

If you are among the 17 million Americans who have diabetes, you are probably working with a doctor to maintain an appropriate treatment program. But what if you could do more to improve your health? In this book, Gene Bruno reveals natural ways to complement your current diabetes management.

The author first explains what complementary therapy means, stressing that the treatments he recommends are meant to enhance your current diabetes program, not replace it. He then defines diabetes and details nutritional modifications that can be helpful in its control. The remainder of the book is devoted to diabetes symptoms and natural methods for dealing with them, as well as important information on potential interactions between prescription drugs and alternative therapies. Unique in its approach, *A Guide to Complementary Treatments for Diabetes* will help you assume an active role in your diabetes program and enjoy the greatest health possible.

$7.95 US • 240 pages • 4 x 7-inch mass paperback • ISBN 978-0-7570-0322-6

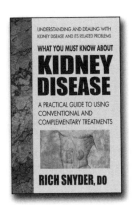

What You Must Know About Kidney Disease

A Practical Guide to Using Conventional and Complementary Treatments

Rich Snyder, DO

What You Must Know About Kidney Disease answers patients' most frequent questions about kidney disease treatment options and provides the up-to-date information needed to cope with this potentially devastating problem. Part I provides an overview of the kidneys' structure and function, Part II examines kidney disorders and their conventional treatments, and Part III provides an in-depth look at the most effective complementary therapies. *What You Must Know About Kidney Disease* will help you understand the challenges ahead and choose the very best treatments available.

$17.95 US • 192 pages • 6 x 9-inch quality paperback • ISBN 978-0-7570-0326-4

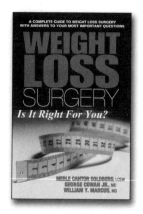

WEIGHT LOSS SURGERY
Is It Right for You?

Merle Cantor Goldberg, LCSW, George Cowan, Jr., MD, and William Y. Marcus, MD

For the thousands of people affected by severe obesity, the decision to undergo weight loss surgery can be a matter of life and death. But it is not a simple procedure, and once done, it produces life-altering changes. To help you make the best possible choice, three experts share their experience, knowledge, and findings about weight loss surgery. Merle Cantor Goldberg is a leading psychotherapist specializing in eating disorders; Drs. Marcus and Cowan have helped develop many of the techniques used in bariatric surgery.

Weight Loss Surgery first addresses important questions about your qualification for this type of surgery, as well as the various options available. It then presents a comprehensive overview of pre-op visits and the post-op recovery period, examining the psychological and physical impacts of surgery.

$17.95 US • 304 pages • 6 x 9-inch quality paperback • ISBN 978-0-7570-0145-1

BITE IT & WRITE IT!
A Guide to Keeping Track of What You Eat & Drink

Stacie Castle, RD, Robyn Cotler, RD, Marni Schefter, RD, and Shana Shapiro, RD

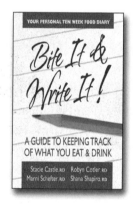

Professionals know that keeping track of what you eat and drink is the most effective way to improve your dietary habits. Designed by four nutritionists who have successfully used this system in their practices, *Bite It & Write It!* combines a structured food journal with an easy-to-follow nutrition guide.

Bite It & Write It! presents ten health goals—one for each week of the journal—and lets you record your daily food consumption as you work toward your objective. To help you along the way, the authors supply a wealth of nutritional information that will empower you to change the way you think about food and make a new commitment to improving your health. With this guide, you can track your calories, carbs, sodium, and water; record exercise; learn how to plan and prepare meals; and navigate restaurant menus without blowing your diet.

$7.95 US • 192 pages • 4 x 7-inch mass paperback • ISBN 978-0-7570-0343-1

For more information about our books, visit our website at www.squareonepublishers.com